Raw
Energy

STEPHANIE TOURLES

124 Raw Food Recipes for
Energy Bars, Smoothies, and Other Snacks
to Supercharge Your Body

Storey Publishing

The mission of Storey Publishing is to serve our customers by
publishing practical information that encourages
personal independence in harmony with the environment.

Edited by Margaret Sutherland and Rebecca Springer
Art direction and book design by Dan O. Williams
Text production by Liseann Karandisecky

Photography by © Kevin Kennefick
Food styling by Frances Duncan and Dan O. Williams

Indexed by Christine Lindemer, Boston Road Communications

Storey Publishing
210 MASS MoCA Way
North Adams, MA 01247
www.storey.com

Printed in China by Toppan Leefung Printing Limited
10 9 8 7 6 5 4 3 2 1

Library of Congress Cataloging-in-Publication Data

Tourles, Stephanie L., 1962–
  Raw energy / Stephanie Tourles.
     p. cm.
  Includes index.
  ISBN 978-1-60342-467-7 (pbk. : alk. paper)
  1. Cookery (Natural foods) 2. Raw food diet.
  3. Vegetarian cookery. 4. Raw foods. I. Title.
TX741.T68 2010
641.5'636—dc22
                    2009028675

CONTENTS

Dedication

To Rick O'Shea IV — the smartest, funniest, most energetic and beautiful dog I've ever been blessed to have share my life. You warmed my heart, my soul, and my feet on cold winter nights, and tested my endurance on our daily, six-mile, Cape Cod seashore walks. I'll never forget the porcupine mishaps and romps through the Maine woods. I'll miss your smiling face and your constant presence in my office when I sit down at the computer to write.

Rest in peace, my furry friend.

August 1, 2008

Acknowledgments

Special gratitude goes out to the folks at Storey Publishing, who have invited me to share my passion for whole, living, raw foods with you, my dear readers. Plus, I'd like to thank the good Lord for the following people who have contributed to my joie de vivre and my knowledge and love of the natural world, organic gardening, and preparation and appreciation of food: Thank you to Phenie Ashe and the late Earl C. Ashe, my grandparents, for teaching me about the goodness of raw, garden-fresh vegetables, wild blackberries, muscadines, and luscious persimmons, and for feeding me scads of thick, juicy, savory tomato sandwiches — my favorite. Thanks for the inheritance of an incredibly green thumb, too!

Thank you to my late grandmother, Grace Anchors, for the pure enjoyment of her moist, tender, flaky, Georgia biscuits, creamy butter beans, and tangy bread-and-butter pickles.

Much gratitude goes to my mother, Brenda Anchors, for ridding our family home of junk food and introducing us to the benefits of whole foods and supplements decades before health food was "in," and to my dad, Mike Anchors, for many lengthy family vacations, delicious outings to authentic French and Mexican restaurants, and exposure to unfamiliar fresh, regional foods. Thanks for filling my mind with knowledge, my youth with experience, and my mouth with exquisite tastes when you could have instead filled our new home with expensive, fancy furniture.

Thank you to my husband, Bill, for building and designing spectacular garden enclosures that are simply works of art. Thanks for making gardening a sheer sensory delight. Your crafting hands are truly blessed, my dear!

Thanks to Nancy Sullivan, my mother-in-law, for teaching me the beauty and necessity of texture and color whether in the home, on the plate, or in the garden. I'm grateful to the late Helen Nearing for the inspiration to eat primarily raw and vegetarian, and to live simply — as close to nature as possible. Thanks to Candis Cantin, my beloved Community Herbalist Program teacher, for continually emphasizing throughout our lessons that our bodies, minds, and spirits become what we eat and assimilate, and that the keys to health are whole foods and herbal nourishment, enjoyment of life and work, sufficient rest, and exercise, combined with good digestion of food and life experiences. So amazingly true. Thank you, Margaret Sutherland of Storey Publishing, editor of *Raw Energy,* for believing in the power of raw foods and understanding my need to relay this message to all of my health-seeking readers.

THE BENEFITS OF RAW SNACKS

Raw Energy was written especially for those of you seeking healthful and dramatically different alternatives to empty-calorie snack foods such as doughnuts, muffins, white-flour bagels, vending machine junk, processed cookies, cakes, candy, crackers, and chips, fast-food milkshakes, artificially flavored milk drinks, and pasteurized canned and bottled juices — not to mention so-called energy bars that frequently contain refined fruit syrups and high-fructose corn syrup.

The methodology of food preparation in *Raw Energy* represents a huge departure from the way most Americans cook. My aim with this book is to introduce you to a new realm of food preparation: uncooking! I hope to educate and make you, my health-conscious readers, aware that raw snacks can be far more satisfying than conventional snacks while providing deep, sustained, "get-up-and-go" power and promoting health, vitality, and good looks — as they tantalize the taste buds. The all-raw-ingredient recipes are easy to make, delicious, and delightful to the eye and palate. And better still, they are highly nutrient-dense and enzymatically potent: raw foods retain their naturally occurring enzymes, which typically make them easier on the digestive system than cooked foods. These *energy treats* consist of real, whole foods, and are completely unheated and uncooked, as is each individual ingredient. Unlike most "no-bake" cookbooks published to date, *Raw Energy* recipes contain no sugar, fruit juice concentrate, jams or jellies, marshmallows or fluff, corn syrup, chocolate syrup, flour, dairy products, refined salt, candy pieces, toasted or roasted ingredients, malt sugar, chocolate or butterscotch chips, sulfured dried fruit, or hydrogenated fats. They *do* contain raw nuts and seeds, raw nut butters, raw unprocessed honey, unsulfured dried fruits and coconut, raw oats, raw carob and raw cocoa (yes, raw cocoa powder does exist), freshly extracted juices, nut milks, and all types of fresh and frozen fruits. I even use raw sweet potatoes and zucchini to create sinfully delicious, crispy, dehydrated vegetable chips. These snacks are good for your body (nutrition and taste), mind (no guilt), and soul (satisfying).

> Raw foods retain their naturally occurring enzymes, which typically make them easier on the digestive system than cooked foods.

What is the real health difference between my raw snacks and ubiquitous commercial snacks? Most conventional snacks are made with processed, refined, nutritionally empty ingredients with a sprinkling of preservatives and synthetic flavorings and a heavy-handed complement of white sugar and sodium. Yes, consuming them will indeed give you a real, albeit temporary, energy lift when you need it most. But because they are not created from whole foods consisting of unprocessed proteins, essential fats, and complex carbohydrates that digest slowly and feed your body with sustained vitamin- and mineral-rich pep, but instead are made of refined ingredients, stripped of their former life-giving elements, they will cause your blood sugar to spike. Within an hour or so, the opposite happens: your blood sugar plummets, and low blood sugar means low energy, a cranky attitude, and a hankering for even more junk. By consistently consuming these types of snack foods, day in and day out, you may have unknowingly jumped into an unhealthy eating cycle replete with unstable energy, a raging appetite, poor health and mood, and a less-than-radiant appearance.

It's time to hop off that merry-go-round of poor snacking choices. The recipes in *Raw Energy* are chock-full of nutrients and long-term energy boosters that taste so incredibly good, you'll wonder why you haven't been snacking this way all along. These raw snacks meet your body's nutrient quota, trigger your natural appetite-regulating hormones, and won't leave you wanting more. We tend not to overeat the foods that satisfy on all levels.

> These raw snacks meet your body's nutrient quota, trigger your natural appetite-regulating hormones, and won't leave you wanting more.

The basic goal of this book is simple: to introduce you to a new way of snacking healthfully in the raw. The snack recipes in this book eliminate the negatives and accentuate the positive aspects of snacking, helping to maximize vigor, vitality, beauty, physical stamina, and endurance at every stage of life. These family- and friend-tested recipes will aid in the achievement of the utmost nature has to offer: total, resilient, whole-body health, with eyes that sparkle, hair that is lustrous, skin that is fresh, glowing, moist, and smooth, nails that are strong, bodily organs that function well and work in harmony with each other, and — best of all benefits, as far as I'm concerned — mental and physical energy to spare. The road to health can be paved with wonderful freshness, new taste sensations, vibrant colors, and delectable flavors that make your taste buds dance and your spirits soar.

Anyone who is still a bit dubious or isn't sure about the taste excitement of whole, raw snack foods will swallow his or her skepticism with the first bite of my Creamy Carob Freezer Fudge or sip of my Papaya Sunset Soup. So turn the pages and absorb a bit of information about the fresh world of raw foods and the importance of regular snacking. Learn how to stock your kitchen with the best raw ingredients and essential food-processing equipment and gadgets, and read the primer on learning how to "uncook." Then jump right in, find a recipe that piques your interest, get your hands messy, and be prepared to enjoy some luscious snacks in the raw. The recipes are relatively simple to concoct, yet exciting on both visual and taste-satisfying levels. Once you get the knack of cooking in the raw, I hope you will be inspired to tap in to your own inner creativity in tweaking these recipes to suit your own personal tastes and dietary needs.

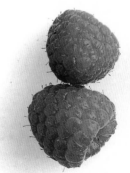

Chapter One

RAW SNACK BASICS

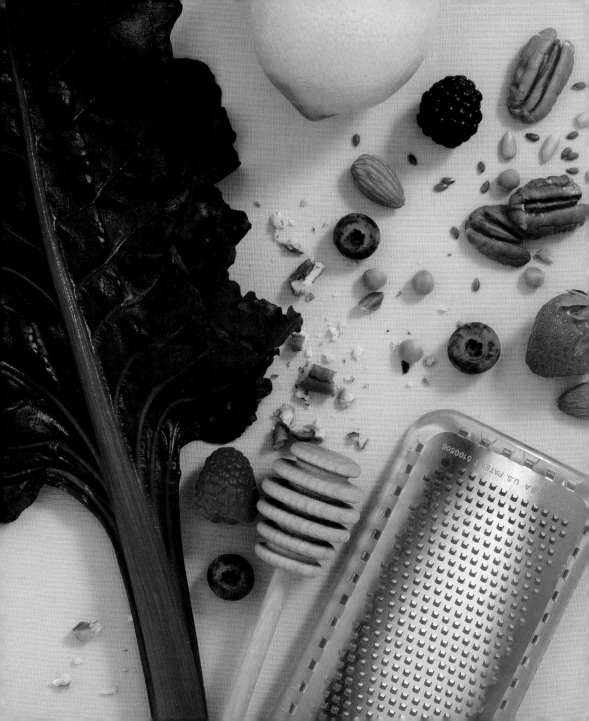

Raw foods are consumed in their purest, most simple form — the way nature serves them up to us. They are real, whole foods that are uncooked, unadulterated, and unprocessed, not refined and stripped of their naturally occurring nutrients. They are never heated above a certain temperature, usually between 95°F and 120°F (35–49°C), as might occur during sun-drying or using a food dehydrator. They rarely come in bottles or jars, and never in cans or aseptic boxes, as processing methods involved in storing foods in these containers require boiling liquids.

The raw foods used in this book are free from chemical preservatives and processing additives; they comprise fresh fruits, vegetables, nuts, seeds, grains, and beans that are wild or organically grown, plus dehydrated, sprouted, and fermented preparations. Also included in this list are raw condiments and nutrition-boosting recipe additions such as dried barley grass and wheatgrass, algae, sea salt, raw apple cider vinegar, herbs, spices, and cold-pressed, unrefined oils.

Raw foods can be prepared by chopping, blending, puréeing, liquefying, slicing, shredding, freezing, dehydrating, or juicing — they just can't be heated to over approximately 120°F (49°C). Don't assume that attempting to include more raw snack foods in your diet is limiting because you can't cook or use cooked ingredients. Far from it! Raw food ingredient combinations are limited only by your imagination. The creative possibilities that exist within the context of raw food snacking are boundless. If simplicity in all things is your motto, you can always satisfy your raw snack cravings with a bunch of sweet grapes, a single juicy nectarine, an avocado drizzled with raspberry vinaigrette, or a crunchy handful of tasty almonds.

The recipes in this book use only animal-product-free ingredients, with the exception of raw honey and bee pollen; these foods are made by living, buzzing creatures. If you are a strict vegan, feel free to omit them and use substitutions such as agave nectar.

So that you know where I'm coming from, let me tell you about my personal eating habits. My current diet is approximately 75 percent vegan, including 60 to 70 percent raw foods. The 25 percent that is not vegan includes a bit of local seafood, farm-fresh eggs, raw goat's milk, and raw goat's milk cheeses. Regarding the raw goat products, I live in a rural town on the Maine coast, where I have access to these wonderful, nutrient- and enzyme-rich, unpasteurized foods. It is legal to purchase them here, so I do enjoy them on a regular basis. I've gotten to know the local small-scale farmers and completely trust their caretaking and production methods. The health and welfare of the animals, the cleanliness of their bedding areas, and sanitation during the milking process are of the utmost importance to me, and should be to you, as well, if you decide to include these types of raw animal foods in your diet.

> Raw food ingredient combinations are limited only by your imagination. The creative possibilities are boundless.

You may not agree with all of my dietary habits, but they satisfy my physical and mental needs at this particular time in my life, and your dietary habits can do the same for you. I feel that the act of eating should be one of pure pleasure; and what one decides to eat, purely personal.

Why Eat Raw?

The nutrient energy derived from the foods consumed in our daily diets shapes, forms, and drives all systems within our bodies. I can't state that fact more simply or accurately. The quality of food consumed is the catalyst that affects one of three end results: a body exhibiting radiant health, beauty, and vitality; a body coasting along through life with mediocre health, appearance, and energy levels; or a body suffering with disease, discomfort, and exhaustion from malnourishment.

Try to fathom the concept that some people, medical professionals included, believe that food does not affect the workings of the human body to any significant degree. How can that be? How can what you drink, eat, digest, and absorb into your very being, your very substance, not play a fundamental role in determining how you function, feel, look, and energetically exist? What you consume — high quality or poor quality — is the fuel that keeps your body going; it affects your individual power, appearance, and well-being.

Right now, I'm going to ask you to read the book title again. Go ahead . . . flip back to the front cover. I want the words *raw energy* to imprint themselves onto your brain. Why? To put it in very simple terms: increased energy intake means increased energy output. Or, in other words, when you consume more whole, nutritionally vibrant, unheated foods, you will invariably boost your body's natural ability to produce, store, and utilize large quantities of expendable energy, thus dramatically improving your mental, physical, and spiritual capabilities.

A diet high in raw foods will *supercharge* your energy level and replenish depleted reserves. Raw foods are easy for most people to digest — digestion being the key to absorption and assimilation of valuable nutrients necessary for copious energy production. Like you, whether I'm working, playing, gardening, or simply going out for a long walk, I want to have plenty of energy to help me accomplish my goals as well as enjoy my leisure time. Foods that are loaded with unheated, unrefined carbohydrates, proteins, and healthful fats will leave your body's cells filled to the brim with fuel for the daily chores of life. They contain the necessary nutritional molecular components that actually power the process of anabolism, or construction of new cells — initiating growth of tissues, repairing existing damage, and replacing aged or inferior cells within your body.

And you will have plenty of energy left over to do those activities you long to do. A beauty bonus: Visible effects from the added dietary nourishment will quickly become noticeable. Your skin, hair, nails, and eyes will glow. I'm promising a lot from the mere addition of raw snack foods to your daily diet, I realize. But it just makes sense that if you eat better, you'll feel better, and you'll ultimately look better, too!

I'm very visual, tactile, and sensual, and I like the fact that working with and eating raw plant foods engages my senses. Raw plant foods are beautiful to look at and uniquely shaped; they offer textures that range from moist and juicy to soft, chewy, and crunchy; they're often brilliantly colored; and they are rich in unbelievable flavors and tantalizing aromas. Because they offer so much in the way of sensory stimulation, raw foods can be enjoyed on every level.

Over the years, I have seen firsthand what a diet rich in whole, raw, unrefined foods can do for your hair, skin, nails, overall health, and energy. Eating this way can take you beyond a lackluster appearance and mediocre health. An increased consumption of raw foods can result in pure radiance and abounding vibrancy, and it can also provide the healing nutrition your body needs to prevent or even reverse some chronic diseases. Because raw foods are generally high in fiber, filling, and full of cell-satisfying nutrition, they can even help with weight loss. All of the reasons I've mentioned above are why I am encouraging you to change your snacking habits. You can truly be at your best if you eat more whole, raw, unadulterated foods.

If you want your joie de vivre to increase, if you want to attract and create health, beauty, and energy in your life, then you have to take control of what you're eating. By increasing the quantity of pure, raw foods in your daily diet, you are actively and positively working toward achieving a higher level of true well-being.

Naturally Occurring Food Enzymes

Since the early years of the twentieth century, there has been a dramatic shift in dietary habits around the world, and particularly in North America. Once we relied on our own gardens or those of our close neighbors to provide us with wholesome, fresh food — food that was frequently raw, sun-dried, fermented, or cultured, minimally processed, and enzyme-rich. This food was chock-full of life-sustaining nutrients and brimming with exquisite taste. But no more. Now we leave the growth and processing of our food primarily to the mega-farmers, those large impersonal corporations that operate with profits and production quotas, rather than our precious health, in mind. For the vast majority of us, this means that we consume a diet high in overcooked, enzyme-deficient, chemically preserved, nutritionally poor, and artificially "enriched" foods. Sadly, this diet also tends to include far too much salty, sugar-laden fast food. In these fast-paced times, health too often takes a backseat to "convenience" when making dietary choices.

Never before have we had more creature comforts yet endured so much physical pain, illness, and general unwellness. Never before have heart disease, diabetes, cancer, obesity, depression, high blood pressure, and other degenerative diseases been as prevalent as they are now.

Organic, raw foods can play a significant role in preventing and even reversing many of these terribly life-disrupting, uncomfortable, and potentially deadly diseases, and the naturally occurring enzymes they contain are the keys to success.

Just what are enzymes? Humbart Santillo, author of *Intuitive Eating* and an expert on raw foods, describes the constructive effects that live enzymes have on health as follows:

> An enzyme is said to be a protein molecule, and each enzyme acts in certain ways in the body doing specific jobs such as digesting food, building protein in the bones and skin, and aiding detoxification, to name a few. Once we cook food at high temperatures, though, the enzyme is destroyed. It no longer carries on its designated function. Although the physical protein molecule is still present, it has lost its life force. Much like a battery that has lost its power, the physical structure remains but the electrical energy which once animated it is no longer present. A protein molecule is actually only the carrier of enzyme activity. In experiments described in *Chemical Reviews* (1933), the activity of one protein molecule was transferred over to another protein substance, leaving the original molecule devoid of its original activity. This only proves further that an enzyme is the invisible activity or energy factor and not just the protein molecule itself. So, for clarity, let us agree that a protein molecule is a carrier of the enzyme activity, much like the light bulb is the carrier for an electrical current.

Life could not exist without enzymes. They are in the cells of every living plant, animal, and human being on earth and are the essential manual

Why Unfired Foods?

Organic, live food is your best Medicare, your ticket to prolonged youth. Nature's foods are in their most nutritious state when eaten raw, picked ripe from orchard or garden. Cooking destroys all enzymes, lecithin, many vitamins and much of the protein. As much as 85 percent of the original nutrients may be lost in cooking.

— Viktoras Kulvinskas, *Love Your Body: Live Food Recipes*

workers, the labor force, for every chemical action and reaction that takes place. We couldn't walk, talk, breathe, digest food, heal, build bone, have a thought, or grow hair without them.

Enzymes are the sparks of life. Let me give you an example: When you eat raw pumpkin or sunflower seeds or almonds, you are ingesting live, enzyme-rich seeds. When planted in moist earth, these little storehouses of nutrient energy will sprout into living plants, capable of maturing and reproducing more edible seeds and nuts. Try this same test with a roasted, baked, or boiled seed or nut — all they will do is rot. They are dead matter. The spark of life has been cooked out of them.

The significant, health-promoting difference between live (raw) and dead food is the enzymatic activity contained within the cells of raw food. All foods untouched by a heat source over 120°F (49°C) have an abundance of enzymes.

Unlike animals in the wild, which live their entire lives on raw foods, man attempts to build healthy cells out of primarily deficient, dead foods that are lacking in live enzymes — much to the detriment of his well-being. When a food is heated, the naturally occurring enzymes become deactivated. Cooking also depletes vitamins, damages proteins and essential fats, and results in the creation of free radicals — major contributors to many diseases, including cancer.

Digestion takes a lot of energy. The process of digestion begins with your digestive tract chemically and mechanically breaking into tiny particles the food you just ate. Then, with the assistance of food enzymes (available in raw food only) and digestive enzymes produced by the salivary glands, stomach, pancreas, liver, gallbladder, and intestines, essential nutrients are extracted and allowed to pass through the minute pores of the intestinal wall into the bloodstream to be transported to and assimilated by your cells and converted into energy or the building materials of nerves, muscles, blood, bones, glands, and more. At the end of the digestive journey, all waste products, including fiber, are evacuated.

Digestive enzymes are vital catalysts, complex molecules that accelerate chemical processes. They are involved in catabolism (breaking down) of larger molecules into the readily absorbable, smaller building blocks that the body requires. When you eat food that has been cooked, your digestive system receives no enzymatic assistance from that food and has to produce all of the enzymes necessary to digest, break down, and process what you consume. It accomplishes this task by calling upon

Enzyme-Rich Plant Foods

The following exceptionally tasty plant foods are noted for their high enzyme content when consumed in raw, unheated form:

avocados	kiwifruit
bananas	lemons
cranberries	mangoes
dates	papayas
extra-virgin olive oil	pineapples
figs	unfiltered raw honey
grapes	

the pancreas, liver, gallbladder, and other organs to contribute enzymatic reserves, stealing the energy of those organs away from other jobs, which can slow the metabolism, compromise the immune system, and leave you feeling less than energetic.

Digestive enzymes and metabolic enzymes (those that keep your arteries clear, run your organs, build healthy tissues, and keep your blood sugar balanced, among other things) aid very different bodily functions, yet they are produced primarily in the same organs — the liver and pancreas. When the body doesn't receive sufficient enzymes to perform its digestive tasks due to a lack of raw, enzyme-packed foods in the daily diet,

Enzymes Are a Component Part of Living Matter

Nature has placed enzymes in food to aid in the digestive process instead of forcing the body's enzymes to do all of the work. It is to be remembered that we inherited an enzyme reserve at birth and this quantity can be decreased as we age by eating an enzyme-deficient diet. By eating most of our food cooked, our digestive systems have to produce all of the enzymes, thus causing an enlargement of the digestive organs. To supply such enzymes, the body draws on its reserve from all organs and tissues, causing a metabolic deficit. If each of us would take in more exogenous enzymes (those enzymes taken from outside sources), our enzyme reserve would not be depleted at such a rapid pace. This would keep our metabolic enzymes more evenly distributed throughout the organism. This is one of the most health-promoting measures that one could implement into his or her daily lifestyle.

— Humbart Santillo, *Intuitive Eating*

these organs slow their pace of creating much needed metabolic enzymes in order to further assist in the digestive process. The manufacturing of digestive enzymes doesn't come without a cost, though. The liver and pancreas require energy to produce additional enzymes, and this energy drain hinders their performance of vital metabolic functions and retards processes of detoxification, fat-burning, and energy production. It has been reported that the majority of Americans are suffering from what is termed "enzyme exhaustion" — and the bloat, weight gain, fatigue, depression, and illnesses that come along with it.

Enzyme-deficient foods do not tend to digest properly, and what isn't digested doesn't nourish you. Improper digestion equals indigestion and putrefaction of food in the stomach. This putrefied material, as it continues its digestive journey, leaves behind a coating on the walls of the small and large intestines, diminishing the absorption of nutrients and impeding the expulsion of toxins through the intestinal wall and the evacuation of wastes from the body. Consistently compromised digestion creates conditions within the body that are ripe for the establishment and multiplication of disease-causing bacteria, fungi, and viruses, thus causing the body to become susceptible to fatigue, infection, and illness. Frequent sufferers of indigestion can often be seen popping multiple antacid pills throughout the day or gulping one of those colorful bottles of nasty-tasting, chalky, gastric-distress-comforting liquids. Those products provide only temporary relief and never get to the root of the problem.

Remember that high enzyme reserves equal high vitality and low enzyme reserves equal low vitality. Your enzyme reserves are drained by eating a diet consisting primarily of cooked foods. A very high level of stress and the overuse of alcohol also adversely affect enzyme production. It is important that the body's enzyme level be preserved, and not depleted, in order to ensure lifelong health and energy.

When consumed and properly chewed, raw food, rich in enzymes, will practically digest itself, without asking the digestive system for assistance over and above the normal call of duty. This leaves you with a surplus of energy to do with what you wish. That's primarily what this book is about — having more energy. Fortunately, raw plant foods taste good and are a delight to eat, so it shouldn't be too difficult to add more of these luscious morsels to your diet.

Why Organic?

Do you really know what you're eating when you bite into a fresh peach, dine on a colorful spinach, walnut, and pear salad with basil vinaigrette, or enjoy a bowl of ripe, plump strawberries with cashew cream for dessert? Do you know where the food came from or how it was grown and processed? Unless you are buying certified organic food from your grocery store, local co-op, farmers' market, or mail-order supplier, you might not like the answer.

Today more than ever, our mass-produced food supply is contaminated with myriad chemicals that have the potential to cause harmful side effects, if not immediately, then in the years ahead. Farmers are applying ever-increasing amounts of synthetic chemicals to crops, virtually poisoning the soil. These unnatural substances kill the naturally occurring microorganisms and worms in the soil that break down organic matter, loosen the soil, and release nutrients for crop uptake. Combine this practice with poor soil management and the resulting soil becomes dead, depleted, compacted, and incapable of growing nutritious food, ultimately requiring even more man-made fertilizers to be spread upon it. The land may be ultimately abandoned and deemed useless, incapable of sustaining growth and life.

Opt for Organically Grown

When you regularly eat conventionally grown produce, many pesticides, herbicides, and other chemicals tend to build up in your body, especially in the fatty tissue. Because the long-term health effects are unknown or unclear, why take that risk? The dozen most contaminated fruits and vegetables are strawberries, apples, bell peppers, cherries, nectarines, peaches, grapes, pears, spinach, celery, raspberries, and potatoes. Especially for this produce, opt for organically grown when you can, and you'll dramatically reduce your exposure to potentially hazardous chemicals. Also, try to reduce or eliminate your intake of imported produce, as some countries use greater concentrations of chemicals than what is allowed in American agriculture.

Until the "health food" movement of the 1960s and the rise of the modern organics movement, most people purchased their groceries at their favorite local supermarket and didn't give it much thought. Food was food, or so many consumers blithely assumed. Well, the tide is rapidly turning on that consensus — finally.

Eating organically is not a newfangled idea, however. It's how most of our grandparents and great-grandparents ate and raised their food before chemical farming "improved" our crops and growing methods. A holistic system of farming — a system of being in harmony with Nature rather than trying to tame or maim her — is the preferred method of all food production. One of the key tenets of organic farming is the belief that sustainable farming practices should mimic nature. Nurture and feed the soil, till it all under, sow seed and grow food, harvest the abundance and share the bounty, sow the proper cover crops, and allow the soil appropriate rest so that it can naturally replenish its stores, and then start all over again. The bounty of the land can feed the humans who farm there and the animals that might live and thrive on it, as well.

I realize, that for many people, eating a diet composed entirely of organically raised food is the ideal, but such foods may not always be available or within reach of your budget. Because the demand for organic food is growing rapidly, it will become more readily available and prices will, in time, come down.

If you want to eat food that is locally produced and organically grown, you will need to do a bit of homework and not just depend on what's labeled "organic" at your supermarket. Do some research and ask around until you find a small-scale, local organic farmer, co-op, or farmers' market that you trust. Get to know the farmers. See where your food comes from, if you can. Perhaps you could join an organic food collective or CSA (Community Supported Agriculture) group where you buy a "share" of a farm and the farmer will deliver fresh produce to you. Try your hand at gardening; growing your own food is a satisfying choice if you have even a small plot of land. It is amazing how much produce you can grow in a small space by utilizing intensive gardening methods.

Reduce Toxic Residues in Your Diet

Recent studies indicate that of all the toxic chemical residues in the American diet, almost all, 95 percent to 99 percent, comes from meat, fish, dairy products, and eggs. If you want to include pesticides in your diet, these are the foods to eat. Fortunately, you can overwhelmingly reduce your intake of these poisons by eating lower on the food chain, and not choosing foods of animal origin.

— John Robbins, *Diet for a New America*

For long-term optimal health, with soundness of body and mind, I recommend eating as much organically grown, supremely high-quality food as your budget will allow. Adding plenty of raw snack foods to your diet is an excellent way to integrate organics on a daily basis. Always strive to eat as close to nature as possible. Your body, mind, spirit, and family will thank you in more ways than you can imagine.

Why Snack?

The recipes in this book will give you 125 delectable reasons to get your snack on! A nutritious, yummy snack can give you a much needed shot of pep during a midmorning or midafternoon energy slump. A snack can satisfy a sweet tooth, help stave off extreme hunger (which will help you to keep your portion sizes in check at mealtime), tide you over if dinnertime is delayed, or even fill in as a meal replacement should you simply be too busy to eat one of your "three squares." A snack can keep your hands busy when trying to quit smoking, cheer you up when you've got the blues, calm an upset child, and be the perfect, light, pre- or post-workout food. Tasty snacks are nice to have on hand to share with friends, family, and unexpected guests, too.

There are times in every day when each of us needs to take a moment to refresh and refuel. This book is all about making the most of those moments, whenever they occur.

Light between-meals snacks can also be quite beneficial if you're watching your waistline. Why? Much of the appetite-stabilizing power of snacks comes from helping to control blood sugar levels. When blood sugar drops too low, you can slip in to "starvation mode" between meals — a physiological signal to your hypothalamus (the appetite center of the brain) that there's no more food coming in and that the body should save its fat stores. If you have a tendency to starve yourself while trying to lose weight or allow yourself to get ravenous between meals, your all-important metabolic rate — or calorie-burning fire — will be dramatically dampened. You want to keep those fires stoked if you're attempting to shed unwanted pounds! Regular intake of whole food (not junk food) snacks will help you burn more calories and keep your appestat (an area of the hypothalamus that controls your appetite for food) satisfied, thus minimizing cravings for super-size meals.

A delicious snack should fully engage the senses and not be mindlessly eaten in haste. It should look good, smell good, taste good, and be good for you. Enjoy a healthful snack as a contribution to the nutrient, energy, beauty, and wellness quota for the day. Snacking should be encouraged, not discouraged, especially if it is full of vital, health-building ingredients.

The Difference Between a Snack and a Meal

Snacks are light bites or sips of energy. They aren't so heavy that they bog you down but are just the right size to get you through a current energy slump or curb those nagging hunger pangs. Raw snacks are yummy mini-meals that can vary in size according to your lifestyle and caloric demands. However you define your snack, one thing's for sure: it's definitely *not* supposed to be an 800-calorie super-size fast-food milkshake or a 600-calorie jumbo box of greasy French fries, nor the caloric equivalent of a full meal that has the potential to slow you down while it digests. A snack should consist of a few tasty bites of nutrient-dense, whole food or a glass of freshly extracted juice or a fruit smoothie that gives you a shot of pep or satisfies a craving, just when you need or desire it most.

Snacking is my preferred way of eating almost all of my meals. I'm a "grazer," and I exist on about six large snacks or light meals per day. This keeps my energy level and metabolism running in high gear and my mind buzzing with creative ideas. If you happen to be a very busy, productive, and active person like me, may I suggest giving my way of eating a try — especially when you are at your busiest and your energy demands are great? You might find yourself pleasantly surprised at your increased physical stamina and mental inspiration.

Tips for Snacking While on the Road

Americans spend a great deal of time behind the wheel — commuting to and from work, doing errands, shuttling the kids to and from school and after-school activities, and traveling. Just because you're out and about and away from the home kitchen, that's no excuse to sabotage your healthful eating habits and scarf down a convenient bag of junk food or hit the drive-through. Instead, try to plan wisely for that inevitable hunger attack. Pack a bag of raw snack goodies such as whole fruit, trail mix, raw brownies, energy bars, date logs, or raw candy, plus an insulated bottle of fresh juice or nut milk and bottles of water before you step foot in the car. Travel "food smart" and be prepared for when hunger strikes — and it will. Balance good nutrition with good taste and always take a wide variety of foods with you so you're less likely to be tempted by one of the local food purveyors of fatty, refined, guilt-laden, high-calorie "pleasures."

Raw Snacks Under 200 Calories

To prevent weight gain and keep energy up and your mood and blood sugar stable, aim for two or three 150- to 250-calorie snacks per day, depending on your activity level. Here are some delicious energy bites and drinks all under 200 calories.

- 2 small celery ribs, each stuffed with 1 tablespoon raw almond butter
- 1 small apple and ¼ cup raisins
- 10 to 15 almonds, hazelnuts, or pecans
- small plate of carrot sticks, bell pepper strips, celery sticks, radishes, and cucumber slices with ⅓ cup guacamole dip
- 2 cups fresh or frozen strawberries or berries drizzled with honey
- 1 cup freshly made almond milk and 1 large dried fig
- quick banana smoothie: ½ frozen banana blended with 1 cup almond milk and dash of cinnamon or nutmeg
- small handful of dried fruit: cherries, apples, apricots, pineapple, or mangoes
- 8-ounce glass of fresh carrot or apple-ginger juice
- ¼ cup of your favorite trail mix
- 2 or 3 small fresh fruit kabobs
- half an avocado with a squeeze of lemon juice and sprinkling of sea salt and dried basil
- 2 cups freshly made gazpacho
- 1 tablespoon raw tahini (sesame butter) or raw almond butter and 1 tablespoon honey swirled together

Snacking on Raw Foods

As I mentioned earlier, my diet currently consists of approximately 60 to 70 percent raw foods, but I didn't reach this level of "rawsome" goodness overnight. I actually began by changing the way I snacked. I'd always tried to eat as healthfully as I could, and, because I'm a holistic esthetician and nutritionist, I knew the beneficial connection that a healthful diet has to looking good and feeling great. It wasn't until I discovered the profound difference that the inclusion in my diet first of raw snack foods, and eventually of more raw foods in general, had on my well-being that I was able to tap in to a potential for wholeness and unbelievable vibrancy I never knew existed. I've always been a naturally energetic person — just ask anyone who knows me — but since I've made the shift from a diet that consisted largely of cooked foods to one that contains a significant percentage of raw foods, you should see me now! Most days I'm practically buzzing, plus my skin has increased moisture — I swear I'm slowly reversing in age — and I'm even healthier than before. What I've experienced isn't unusual; in fact, it's the norm for devoted "raw-foodists."

My days are filled with writing, teaching, working on my herbal and nutritional research and ongoing studies, gardening, and exercising, and I prefer to stay busy most of the time. I thrive on accomplishment and am grateful for a career that I enjoy. In order to sustain all of this activity, I depend on the energy stores I acquire by eating a diet high in raw foods, and that includes plenty of my favorite scrumptious raw snacks. This inner wellspring of dynamic force enables me to enjoy my life in the manner I choose — and I definitely need plenty of go-go juice!

Just about everyone I know has a busy or even hectic lifestyle and a consequent need for unlimited energy. No matter what your daily energy requirements are, everyone needs relatively quick and nutritious, yet taste-indulgent, "pick-me-up" foods that can be eaten at any time of the day — minus that lingering guilty feeling that often accompanies the consumption of standard *snack crap* (pardon my honesty).

This is where the advantages of eating raw, high-energy snacks come into play. The snacks in this book are made from real, energy-boosting, good-for-you, pure food — pure fuel. The raw nuts, fruits, vegetables, grains, seeds, herbs, oils, and sweeteners have nothing added and nothing taken away. My recipes will show you how to combine these ingredients in unique ways to produce snacks with high visual appeal, tantalizing mouthfeel, and lip-smacking lusciousness.

If you still need convincing, here are a few of the many advantages to eating this way.

- *Raw snacks are nutritionally dense.* They truly fill you up and quickly curb hunger because the nutrients are whole, unprocessed, and easily absorbable.

- *Raw snacks are quick to prepare.* Whole fruits, vegetables, nuts, and seeds are nature's original fast-food snacks. For something a bit more involved than a simple piece of fruit, many of my raw snack recipes can be prepared in quantity ahead of time so that they are ready to grab and go.

- *Raw snacks are portable.* Many of these recipes can be stashed in your purse, briefcase, gym bag, or backpack or poured into an insulated bottle for enjoyment later in the day.

- *Raw snacks are always guaranteed fresh.* Unlike most processed, preserved snack foods, raw snacks have not been sitting around on a shelf for an unknown amount of time, rapidly approaching their expiration date.

- *Raw snacks give you peace of mind.* With raw snacks that you make at home, there are no labels to decipher. You *know* what you are sinking your teeth into. You don't need to look out for pesky trans fats, preservatives, high-fructose corn syrup, artificial dyes, refined flour, salt, sugar, or synthetic vitamins or flavorings.

- *Raw snacks are good for the environment.* No energy is required to heat the food, other than a low-heat-output dehydrator for a few recipes. No disposable packaging is required; portable energy bars, trail mixes, vegetable chips, and confections can be stored and transported in reusable containers. No animals are harmed in the production of raw snacks, and no rain forests are cut down to make grazing pasture for livestock. And, finally, no artificial coloring, preservatives, or flavorings are added, which can find their way into our waterways during the manufacture and processing of many commercial snack foods.

Snacking and the Elderly

Healthful snacking can play an integral part in the diets of those over 70. Many older adults simply don't consume enough calories to receive the nutrients they need to feel and function at their best. Reasons for eating less can include illness, physical decline, limited financial resources, diminished appetite due to side effects from medication, loss of taste-bud sensitivity, and social factors such as living alone and stressful living arrangements. Elderly folks who consume two or three quality nutritional snacks throughout the day benefit significantly from higher numbers of calories along with resulting better health, stable blood sugar levels, increased metabolism, and bodily warmth. Be a good Samaritan and check in on your elderly neighbors. I'm sure they'd appreciate a batch of tasty raw snacks or a quart of fresh juice delivered with a smile and bit of friendly conversation.

How to Make Snacking Part of Your Active Day

Light snacks or mini-meals can help to keep you going whether at work, at home, traveling, or before or after a workout, and there are plenty of easy ways to make snacking work for you. Here are some tips for incorporating healthful snacks into your active lifestyle:

- *Make a snack date.* Snack with a friend, coworker, or even your significant other. It's easier to stick to your healthful snacking goals if you have a snack buddy who's trying to do the same, and snacking with a partner gives you time out of your busy day to chitchat and catch up.
- *Have snacks readily available.* When those stomach rumblings start to get the better of your willpower, reach for a snack in your purse, gym bag, or desk drawer.
- *Snack for refreshment and refueling.* Be sure to eat a small snack every few hours to help maintain energy and keep your blood sugar level stable.
- *Don't forget fresh juice and smoothies.* A small glass of fruit or vegetable juice or a fruit smoothie makes a light, refreshing snack with instant pep-power. Those natural sugars go right into your bloodstream, providing some quick zippity-zoom. Make your delicious drink in the morning and pack it in an insulated bottle so it's ready when you are.
- *Use a snack as a meal replacement.* No time for breakfast, lunch, or dinner? Substitute a substantial snack (approximately 300 to 600 calories) that includes a good mix of carbohydrates, fats, and proteins

for staying power. Try a couple of raw energy bars, a large portion of trail mix, dehydrated vegetable chips and sesame tahini dip, or a strawberry smoothie made with almond or walnut milk, honey, and a handful of raw oats along with a few whole almonds or walnuts.

- *Pack snacks to go.* Always keep snacks in your car for yourself, your kids, and unexpected travel companions. Apples, grapes, baby carrots, and a zesty sunflower and pumpkin seed blend are great choices. I particularly like to carry around a few Almond-Raisin Cocoa Bites (page 159) . . . so sweet, dense, and yummy!

- *Savor an evening sweet treat.* After dinner, treat yourself to a sweet snack such as a few dried figs, a small plate of apple slices spread with raw almond butter, sprinkled with coconut shreds and drizzled with honey, or one of my favorites — Sesame Calcium Chews (page 239). These three snacks are loaded with calcium and magnesium — the minerals that help build bones, relax your muscles, and encourage sound sleep. Enjoying one of these light, sweet, and healthful snacks is the perfect way to end your busy day and ease into your evening deliciously.

Eat Real Food

Stuff your grandmother would have recognized as food. Stuff that usually doesn't come in a package . . . Real food — whole food with minimal processing — contains a virtual pharmacy of nutrients, phytochemicals, enzymes, vitamins, minerals, antioxidants, anti-inflammatories, and healthful fats, and can keep you alive and thriving into your tenth decade. And remember, *how* you eat is as important as *what* you eat. Mindfulness and consciousness in eating — like in everything else in life — contribute to health and well-being.
— Jonny Bowden, *The 150 Healthiest Foods on Earth*

Use Snacks to Increase Your Energy

Energy is vital. Energy exhibits itself as power, vigor, might, endurance, and vibrancy. Along with oxygen and water, we need large amounts of energy to get through our hectic schedules and deal with the demands of modern life, plus abundant energy left over to do the things we enjoy most — play with our kids, walk the dog, jog on the beach, hike up a majestic mountain, run a marathon, or write that best-selling novel during the wee hours of the morning.

Sadly, though, most of us don't have nearly enough of this precious resource. If you enjoy an active life and participate in regular exercise or sports as part of your daily routine, then having long-term power, strength, and stamina really means a lot. That's where raw, whole-food snacks come into play. *Raw Energy* is an eye-opening look into the world of sustenance snack foods that are unadulterated, nutrient-rich, and easily

Is It Really Hunger or Are You Simply Dehydrated?

Do you find yourself snacking more frequently than you should? Many times what is perceived as hunger is really just thirst in disguise. Try this simple test to determine if you are truly hungry. If you've been snacking healthfully and catch yourself wanting to snack too often, try drinking a big glass of water first, before you reach for another bite. It could be that your body is really dehydrated and crying out for water. This can easily occur if you are particularly active, the weather is warm, or the humidity level is low.

digested and assimilated into your bloodstream. They produce energy reserves to draw from when you need them most but will not weigh you down. Regularly consuming raw snacks will supercharge your body.

Natural energy, or *organic energy,* as I like to call it, derived from an extremely healthful, varied, whole-food diet, tends to be fortifying, potent, consistently present, and balanced. On the flip side, *artificial energy,* or energy derived from refined foods and caffeinated drinks, provides quick stimulation but the energy is fleeting, leaving your fuel tank running on fumes and your zippiness zapped. All exercise and sports enthusiasts know what it feels like to run out of zest. If it happens at the end of your game, competition, or exercise time, that's okay. Then you know you've given it your all. But if your energy balloon deflates midevent, that's no good. Something's amiss.

Real, live, raw-food snacks, in addition to an overall healthful diet and lifestyle, will assist your body in creating the invigorating force sought by every mentally and physically active individual, whether an athlete, busy mom, teenager, construction worker, schoolteacher, executive, landscaper, or student. It is my hope that the snack recipes in this book will help you to reach your goal of fully charging, vitalizing, and energizing your body so that you can wholly and mindfully participate in all that life dishes up to you.

> The destiny of ordinary people and nations
> is decided in the kitchen.
>
> — Bernard Jensen

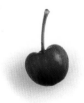

Chapter 2

THE RAW SNACK PANTRY & KITCHEN EQUIPMENT ESSENTIALS

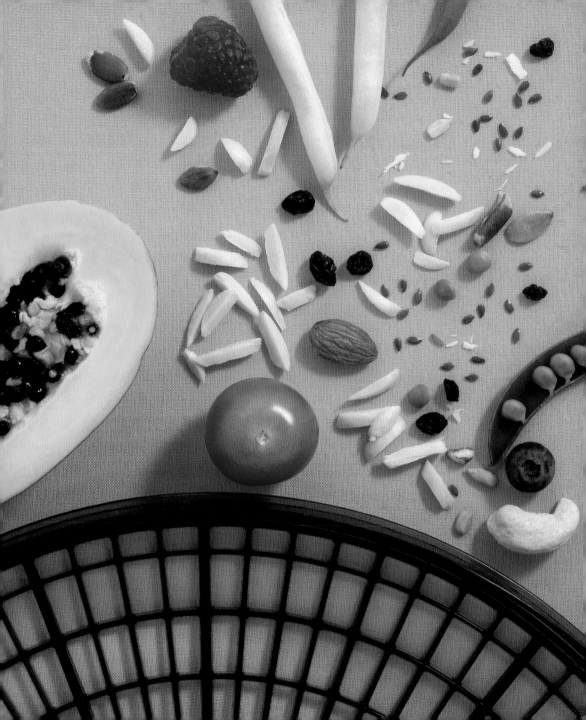

Raw Energy is an introductory manual into the world of raw snack foods. I kept simplicity and familiarity of ingredients and kitchen equipment in mind when creating the recipes. Most of the foods, condiments, herbs, and spices are relatively easy to find and shouldn't be totally foreign to you. Yes, there are those items such as spirulina powder, raw nut butters, bee pollen, mulberries, and carob that some of you may never have even heard of, much less tasted, but that's where the fun lies — in experimentation of new tastes, textures, and aromas.

The Kitchen Essentials equipment list is what I like to call "advanced basic." Almost every appliance and gadget should be familiar — especially if you are a vegan or vegetarian "foodie" and really love to spend time in the kitchen concocting various delicious delights. If you're less experienced in the kitchen, some implements, such as a mandoline, spiral slicer, food dehydrator, juicer, and nut milk bag, will be new to you. Not to worry. I'll explain in detail what each piece does and when to use it to get the most enjoyment and aesthetic pleasure from your foods.

Just where do you find all of the ingredients and kitchen equipment? If you have room for a garden, grow as much organic food as you can. Fresh is always best! Most of the ingredients and even some unique equipment can also be purchased from supermarkets that cater to a health-conscious customer. These stores frequently carry a large variety of organically produced food, which is what I strongly recommend when available. Also try local farmers' markets, co-ops, and smaller health food stores for fresh produce, raw nuts, seeds, nut butters, and organic condiments, herbs, and spices. Most of the equipment can easily be found in kitchen specialty stores.

If you're having no luck in finding what you need within a short driving distance or are simply interested in what else might be available for the raw snack connoisseur, you can also check the Resources section (page 265) for a listing of raw food and kitchen equipment mail-order purveyors and pertinent Web sites.

Get to know your ingredients, kitchen appliances, and gadgets. They are your tools for a rejuvenated, renewed, revitalized, radiant, energetic you. Included in each description below is valuable information — read it, learn it, and absorb it, and use this compendium as a reference guide as you create and concoct your raw energy bars, parfaits, shakes, trail mixes, vegetable chips, and other healthful raw-snack goodies.

Allergies, Food Sensitivities, and Raw Food Safety

The recipes in this book do not include any raw animal products (dairy, eggs, seafood, meat, or poultry) so there is no need to concern yourself about food safety in that context. My recipes do contain plenty of raw fruits, vegetables, nuts, seeds, sweeteners, oils, cocoa, grains, green food powders, seasonings, flavorings, and occasionally roasted peanut butter. If you have any known food sensitivities or allergies, use common sense and avoid any ingredients that can potentially cause discomfort or illness. Allergic reactions to nuts are on the rise these days, and I use a lot of nuts, nut butters, and nut milks in these recipes, so please be extremely careful if these foods are a problem for you. Also remember, *no honey* for infants under the age of one year. Always purchase only the freshest raw ingredients available, store accordingly, wash produce carefully, and use ingredients before they naturally expire.

Raw Snack Pantry Ingredients

Following is an extensive list of almost all of the ingredients I use in my snack recipes. I'm not suggesting that you must have every ingredient in your kitchen in order to enjoy more raw snacks in your diet. I certainly don't have everything on hand every day, but I do try always to have a supply of my favorite raw-snack staples, such as frozen raspberries and strawberries, raisins, dates, dried figs, almonds and pecans, almond butter, tahini, honey, cocoa, and freshly prepared almond milk — all raw, of course. I also keep a fresh assortment of fruits and vegetables readily available in every season.

Your store of ingredients will grow over time as you experiment and become a fan of raw treats. You will develop your own list of favorite ingredients and will want to keep an ample stash on hand for healthful, impromptu snacking.

Water in Recipes

As you will see listed in my recipes, I specify the use of *purified water*. Purified or pure water has minimal flavor, is essential to life and health, and is devoid of man-made chemicals, bacteria, fungi, pollutants, and heavy metals. You can use your favorite bottled water, filtered water, spring water, or distilled water in these recipes. Tap water is not recommended unless you first filter it yourself.

How Do I Know If a Food Is Raw?

With some foods, such as fresh fruits and vegetables, rawness is obvious. When purchasing other ingredients, such as nuts, seeds, nut or seed butters, grains, honey, agave nectar, vinegar, soy sauce, carob, and cocoa, it may not be so obvious, especially if you are unfamiliar with "all things raw." Simply make sure that the label has the word *raw* on it; otherwise it is *not*! If the word *roasted, dry-roasted, toasted, cooked,* or *baked* appears on the label, avoid it. Dried herbs and spices, dried fruits and vegetables, bee pollen, nutritional yeast, and green drink powders are generally considered raw ingredients unless labeled otherwise.

Nuts, Seeds, and Nut and Seed Butters

Other than great taste, nuts, seeds, and nut and seed butters have one thing in common — a high energy value. Nutritionists use this term to indicate that a food is extremely nutrient-dense. Raw nuts and seeds and the butters made from them contain copious quantities of good-for-you fats; are moderate in protein, carbohydrates, and fiber; and are low in sodium. Super-fresh nuts and seeds are chock-full of vitamin E and have generous complements of the B vitamins and important minerals such as calcium, potassium, phosphorus, magnesium, manganese, selenium, copper, iron, and zinc.

When purchasing nuts and seeds, whether buying them shelled or unshelled, they should feel heavy for their size. When biting into them, they should have a nice, fresh snap and slightly sweet taste. Prior to consuming any nuts and seeds, always check for signs of mold, dark spots, or a shriveled appearance, which can indicate poor storage conditions, rot, lack of moisture, or rancidity.

Nuts, seeds, and their butters are perishable and prone to spoilage if not stored properly. They are highly nutritious and can be a bit on the expensive side, so please safeguard your grocery investment. I recommend storing all raw nuts and seeds in the refrigerator or freezer in tightly sealed freezer bags. Raw nut and seed butters purchased in factory-sealed jars can be stored in a cool, dark cupboard until opened, then kept in the refrigerator for a couple of months. If you buy butters such as almond, sunflower seed, or sesame seed paste (tahini), ground fresh and found in the refrigerator case at the health food store, then store them in your refrigerator immediately when you arrive home.

Natural Foods Come in All Shapes and Sizes

You will see that raw (fresh or dried) ingredients such as fruits, nuts, seeds, grains, vegetables, and herbs vary in shape, texture, and size. Due to these variances or natural discrepancies, it is difficult at times to measure ingredients exactly. When making a recipe, your measurements should be as close as possible to what is indicated in the ingredient list, but don't worry if they aren't absolutely perfect. The result will still be delicious.

ALMONDS. These nuts are a universal favorite with a mild, familiar flavor. The versatile almond can be incorporated into so many recipes ranging from creamy almond milk to energy bars. This delicious nut is a good source of easily absorbable vitamins B and E, calcium, potassium, phosphorus, manganese, magnesium, iron, and zinc.

ALMOND BUTTER. My favorite raw substitute for peanut butter is both an instant snack eaten straight off the spoon and a recipe ingredient. Most commercially available almond butter, either freshly ground and refrigerated or processed and sold in jars, is made from roasted almonds, so please make sure that the words *raw almond butter* appear on the label. Fresh almond butter can also be made at home if you have a powerful juicer with a nut butter attachment. Almond butter can be smeared or drizzled on just about everything and even included in thick shakes. Keep raw almond butter in the refrigerator for maximum freshness.

BRAZIL NUTS. These hard, distinctively flavored nuts are one of the best food sources of the trace mineral selenium, which is often deficient in the American diet due to our depleted soils. One of the most calorically dense nuts, Brazil nuts are high in heart-healthy monounsaturated fat and also a good source of vitamins B and E, copper, calcium, zinc, iron, phosphorus, magnesium, and potassium. Brazil nuts can be enjoyed as a simple snack by the handful or added to trail mix or energy bar recipes.

CASHEWS. Everyone loves cashews! These curly nuts, with a generous percentage of heart-healthy monounsaturated fat, B vitamins, potassium, phosphorus, copper, selenium, magnesium, iron, and zinc, make a great snack eaten right out of the bag. Higher in carbohydrates and a little sweeter than other nuts, their softly crunchy texture goes well in many snack recipes. Try them as toppings on parfaits and in muesli, trail mix, raw candy, vegetable dip, and shake recipes.

CASHEW BUTTER. Velvety smooth and mild, cashew butter can be quite expensive, but because these nuts have a relatively soft texture compared to the other nuts, it's easy to make your own ultra-creamy cashew butter in the blender (see recipe for Sweet Cashew Butter Drizzle on page 190). Cashew butter doesn't have a potent flavor of its own, so it blends well with just about every other food and also absorbs flavors beautifully, especially the flavors of apples, citrus fruits, onions, garlic, dates, figs, and cinnamon. It makes fantastic vegan "whipped cream" and fruit drizzles. It also thickens shakes and makes a great base for a vegetable onion dip.

COCONUT. When purchasing coconut, look for unsweetened, dried, raw flakes or shreds. If you have access to fresh, inexpensive coconuts and don't mind the effort of extracting the milk and meat inside, then by all means use them in your raw snack recipes. A star player in energy bites, bars, and balls, dried coconut, with its plentiful supply of fiber and potassium, can be deliciously added to more than half of the recipes in this book.

HAZELNUTS. The hazelnut — also called a filbert — is a good source of calcium, potassium, magnesium, manganese, phosphorus, iron, zinc, copper, and vitamins B and E. This crunchy, uniquely flavored round nut is delicious in energy bars, raw candy, and trail mix recipes. When coarsely ground, it also makes a good crunchy coating on frozen banana slices.

PEANUT BUTTER. Peanut butter is not a raw ingredient, nor is it available raw. Raw peanuts cannot be ground into a spreadable, creamy nut butter. Instead, the end result is very granular and "green" tasting. This is one of two ingredients listed that are exceptions to my all-raw rule (the other being maple syrup). So why include it here? Because it is very familiar to everyone, young and old. If you are trying to convince your spouse, child, or anyone else for that matter to eat more raw snack foods and the only way to coerce them is to smear roasted peanut butter on bananas, carrots, apple or pear slices, or celery sticks, or to blend it with dried fruit and coconut and make raw energy balls or candy, or to make a peanut butter, honey, and almond milk shake, then by all means let them eat peanut butter. Most of the snack will be raw, and peanut butter is a pretty good source of immune-system-enhancing antioxidants, protein, healthful fat, fiber, potassium, calcium, copper, magnesium, manganese, phosphorus, zinc, iron, and B and E vitamins. You can always introduce someone to the other raw nut and seed butters later. Remember, when adding new foods to anyone's diet, including your own, always take baby steps.

PECANS. I grew up in Georgia and Texas — the largest producers of pecans in the United States — and believe me, I've enjoyed my fair share of these quintessentially southern nuts. When super-fresh, these sweet, succulent, plump, oily nuts are my all-time favorites. They add an elegant beauty and exquisite taste to trail-mix, parfait, energy bar, muesli, and confection recipes and are loaded with heart-healthy monounsaturated fat plus potassium, manganese, zinc, phosphorus, magnesium, and vitamins B and E. Raw pecan confections are a truly indulgent snack that just happens to be fabulously flavorful and oh-so-good for you.

PINE NUTS. Also known as *piñons* or *pignoli*, these teardrop-shaped, tiny, pale golden white seeds come from the very large pinecones of the piñon tree. They have a unique, smooth, oily flavor and a bite that is chewy-crunchy and are especially high in protein plus healthful fat, iron, zinc, potassium, magnesium, and the B vitamins. Pine nuts add wonderful flavor, creaminess, and texture to muesli, raw candy, vegan "cheese" spreads, pesto, and energy bar recipes.

PISTACHIOS. The raw pistachio nut is green, not dyed red. I use these little nuts primarily in muesli, parfait, and trail mix recipes to add extraordinary taste, color, and crunch. They're a wonderful source of vitamins B and E, plus iron, phosphorus, potassium, and calcium, and an excellent source of protein.

PUMPKIN SEEDS. Commonly called *pepitas,* these little seeds are a terrific source of phosphorus, selenium, potassium, iron, magnesium, manganese, zinc, protein, and omega-3 fatty acids. A popular snack food by themselves, they're often added to trail mixes for their crunch factor. Try my Pepita and Sunflower Crunchies recipe (page 175) — a wonderful food blend for travel and hiking.

SESAME SEEDS. High in copper, zinc, calcium, magnesium, manganese, potassium, iron, phosphorus, and fiber, sesame seeds also contain vitamins B and E and more protein by weight than any other seed or nut. I use them primarily when making raw candy such as halvah. Try my Sesame Calcium Chews (page 239), a nutritional powerhouse candy that fortifies the body while calming the nerves.

SESAME SEED PASTE. Commonly referred to as *tahini,* sesame seed paste offers a smooth texture with a strong sesame flavor. I use it in raw candy and vegetable dip recipes. Most commercially available tahini, either freshly ground and refrigerated or processed and sold in jars or cans, is made from toasted sesame seeds, so be sure that the words *raw tahini* or *raw sesame seed butter/paste* appear on the label.

SUNFLOWER SEEDS. Universally enjoyed by all, I add sunflower seeds whole or ground to all kinds of recipes. They also make a terrific vegan "cheese" spread. Sunflower seeds are an excellent source of calcium, copper, selenium, potassium, phosphorus, magnesium, iron, zinc, manganese, vitamins B, D, E, and K, and fiber. Combined with pumpkin seeds, they form the "dynamic duo" of snack food blends and provide a rich source of easily assimilated, plant-derived protein — richer than most meats, in fact.

WALNUTS. With a similar nutrient profile to cold-water fatty fish, walnuts are the best available vegetarian "brain food." Walnut meat even looks like the human brain with all of its nooks and crannies! They contain the highest amounts of omega-3 fats of any nut and are a good source of the B vitamins, potassium, phosphorus, manganese, and magnesium, plus lesser amounts of calcium, iron, zinc, and copper. Common English walnuts star in many of my recipes, ranging from raw walnut brownies to delightfully creamy walnut milk. The black walnut, with its richer, more potent flavor, can also be used, but it tends to be difficult to find these days.

Walnuts: A Great Snack for Kids

Several studies have demonstrated greater attention, reduction in behavioral problems, and less "ADD-like" behaviors in school kids when they're given omega-3s. Since it's hard to get kids to eat fish, let alone carry it to school in their lunchbox, walnuts are a really smart idea for a kid snack.

— Jonny Bowden, *The 150 Healthiest Foods on Earth*

Grains

Most raw grains can be difficult to digest unless sprouted. Raw oats and wheat germ are exceptions that I love to use in raw snack recipes due to their versatility and flavor. They are considered complex carbohydrates, and they help keep your energy level on an even keel because they stabilize your blood sugar. These foods have staying power and make powerful breakfast and potent snack ingredients.

OAT GROATS. What the heck is a *groat*? It's the whole oat grain with the outer hull removed, delivering a chewy texture and mild flavor that shines in muesli and parfait recipes. Oats provide B vitamins, potassium, phosphorus, zinc, selenium, manganese, magnesium, and iron, slow-release carbohydrates, and a moderate amount of protein. They are also a great source of soluble and insoluble fiber.

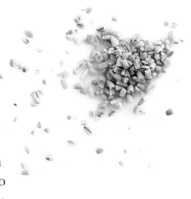

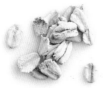

OATS, ROLLED. Everyone is familiar with rolled oats or "oatmeal flakes." Contrary to popular belief, most often these are not raw, but are the result of steaming the whole groat, which is then rolled flat into flakes and dried. Raw oat flakes are available if you seek them out. Remember to look for the word *raw* on the label just to make sure you're getting the real thing. Raw rolled oats are useful in all kinds of recipes that need a starchy binding and good chew, such as in energy bars and balls, raw confections, trail mixes, muesli, and parfaits.

WHEAT GERM. Wheat germ is the heart of the wheat kernel. It is what remains after the outer husk, bran, and endosperm have been removed during processing. Though it represents less than 5 percent of the wheat berry, nutritionally it is a powerhouse, rich in many minerals, fiber, B vitamins, protein, healthful fat, and the antioxidant vitamin E. I like it for its rich, nutty flavor and add it to just about everything except vegetable dishes, juices, and raw soups. When purchasing raw wheat germ, it should be found only in the refrigerated or freezer section of the store, as it becomes rancid quickly. If you find it on a shelf at room temperature, pass it by — more than likely, it's spoiled.

Sweeteners

With the exception of maple syrup, the following sweetening agents have not been refined — their naturally occurring vitamins, minerals, and enzymes are still intact. But, because these natural sweeteners consist primarily of simple sugars that are absorbed rapidly into the bloodstream (agave nectar being the exception), they should be treated with respect and not abused. Use them as you would any other sweetening agent — judiciously — just to add a sweet taste sensation.

AGAVE NECTAR. This natural sweetener is derived from the agave cactus, native to Mexico and the same plant used in the manufacture of tequila. The mildly flavored light amber syrup is 1¼ times sweeter than sugar and thinner than honey but with a very low glycemic index, which makes it an excellent choice for anyone watching his or her reactive carbohydrate intake or suffering from blood sugar disorders such as diabetes. Agave and raw honey can be used almost interchangeably. Be sure the label says *raw* — if it does not, the syrup was heated above 118°F (48°C) during the extraction process and the valuable enzymes have been destroyed.

HONEY. When I was a little girl, my grandfather maintained a few beehives on his farm in northern Georgia. The sourwood honey he harvested from those hives every year was very pale amber in color, almost golden-clear some years. Liquid ambrosia! Food for the gods, I'd say! Sometimes he'd hand me a fresh pint and I'd plop right down and immediately eat nearly half of it with a spoon, honeycomb and all. Doesn't get any better than that!

Most, if not all, of the honey available in the grocery store has been heated and filtered; stay away from that. It *must* say *raw* on the label. A tip-off? Honey that has been heated will remain liquid for a long time, until it eventually thickens and crystallizes. Raw honey will become very thick or slightly hard and crystallized within a few months of being removed from the hive, the exceptions being honies derived from sourwood and tupelo trees, which will remain relatively liquid for a year or more. Look for honey that is raw and unfiltered, complete with tiny specks of pollen, propolis, and beeswax throughout. Ultra high in valuable enzymes, with small amounts of the B vitamins, calcium, iron, copper, manganese, magnesium, potassium, phosphorus, and zinc, honey is a quick energizer due to its high natural sugar content. I use it almost daily to sweeten tea and shakes, drizzle over fruit, and add to raw candy. Because it contains antiviral and antibacterial properties, I even apply it to cuts, scratches, and bug bites to aid in healing.

Honey and Athletic Endurance

All serious athletes — nutrition- and performance-conscious individuals — are aware that the consumption of carbohydrates prior to, during, and after exercise is essential for improved speed, stamina, and muscle recovery. Raw, unprocessed honey, a complex whole food, provides 17 grams of carbohydrates per tablespoon, is high in potassium, tastes great, and is probably the best natural source of energy available to humans due to its near pure sugar content, which is very easily assimilated by the body. Honey can be used as an inexpensive, effective, and more nutritious alternative to commercial sports gels.

MAPLE SYRUP. Definitely not a raw ingredient, maple syrup is made in the spring of the year by tapping or extracting the sap or watery sugar from maple trees in New England and Canada. The raw sap is then boiled down for many hours to reduce water content, which results in a sweet, golden brown syrup that is commonly poured on pancakes and used as a cooking ingredient. Maple syrup is one of two ingredients included in this book that are exceptions to my all-raw rule. So why do I include it? As with peanut butter, it offers a familiar, unique flavor that is adored by most everyone, young and old alike. If the only way to get your family and friends to eat more raw snacks is to substitute maple syrup for the suggested raw sweetener in the recipe, then by all means use it. Over time, they will realize that your raw snacks are yummy and want to try the other raw sweeteners. I'll say it again — and it bears repeating — when introducing new tastes and textures, always take baby steps!

Fruits: Fresh, Dried, and Frozen

All fruits contain an abundance of vitamins, minerals, enzymes, fiber, and natural sugars. Fresh, they are nature's thirst-quenching, naturally sweet, liquid-filled energy foods. The best-tasting fruit is purchased in season and locally from farmers' markets and co-ops. Try to buy organic when available. The freshest fruits make the best juices, smoothies, shakes, and raw fruit soups.

I like to use dried fruit for the intense flavor, sweetening properties, and unique textures it has to offer whether eaten alone or combined into recipes. When purchasing dried fruit, look for unsulfured varieties. They will tend to be darker in color and firmer, slightly drier, chewier, or crunchier than their brighter-colored, moister, softer-textured, sulfured cousins and will taste slightly different. Sulfur dioxide is commonly used on dried fruit, among other things, as a bactericide, disinfecting agent, and preservative. It is not necessary and best avoided. Individuals who are sensitive to sulfur may have asthmalike symptoms after ingestion of this chemical.

Frozen fruits are the main ingredients in my frosty shakes. Bags of organic frozen fruits are available these days from most large supermarkets. When in season, you can also clean, cut, and freeze your own fresh fruit in heavy freezer bags or plastic tubs. That's what I generally do. Frozen fruit allows you to taste summertime in January, at much better quality than the pale, imported specimens available out of season. Frozen fruit is generally picked at the peak of ripeness, for better taste and nutrition. Conveniently no-prep, you can use frozen fruit right from the bag with no peeling or cutting.

Many fruits, such as peaches, strawberries, red raspberries, blackberries, mangoes, cherries, blueberries, and even melons, can be purchased frozen and still retain their luscious, fresh flavors. Frozen pineapple is a little dry, but you may like it, if you can find it. The cost of frozen fruit can be on a par with or even less expensive than fresh fruit.

Wash Before You Eat

The need to wash well applies not only to your hands but also to your fresh fruits and vegetables. You don't always know the details of how they were grown, the route they've traveled, or who's handled them — not even the organic ones. So, please, for safety's sake, wash all produce thoroughly to remove dust, animal dander, mold, bacteria, and pesticide residue with a nontoxic, biodegradable soap and rinse well prior to consumption.

APPLES. A rich source of sugars and fiber, particularly if eaten with the peel, apples also contain a healthy dose of antioxidant flavonoids, boron, potassium, and small amounts of vitamins B and C. Tart, firm apples go through the juicer with greater ease than softer-fleshed apples. Fresh apple slices also make tasty snacks when slathered with fresh almond or cashew butter. Dried apples can be added to muesli, trail-mix, and fruit compote recipes.

APRICOTS. Particularly rich in antioxidant carotenoids and flavonoids, apricots also provide potassium and vitamin C and are an excellent source of iron and calcium when eaten in dried form. Dried Turkish apricots add a pleasantly sweet taste and chewy texture to energy bars, trail mixes, fruit compotes, muesli, and raw candy. My recipes call for dried, unsulfured apricots exclusively, as fresh apricots are particularly perishable, and the supermarket specimens are rarely worth eating, even during their short season.

BANANAS. This versatile, sweet, filling fruit provides significant amounts of energizing carbohydrates (sugars), potassium, and moderate amounts of vitamins B and C. I like to use fresh, creamy ripe bananas in parfaits. Dried bananas can be eaten alone as leathery fruit bites and also added to chewy raw candy.

A freezer bag full of frozen bananas comes in handy for impromptu smoothies, shakes, and frozen fruit creams. When fruits begin to get speckled and slightly soft but not overripe, black, or mushy, peel bananas, put them in a plastic freezer bag (either whole bananas or broken in half), and freeze for up to 2 months.

BLACKBERRIES. As a child, one of my favorite desserts was my grandmother Ashe's fresh blackberry pie complete with a thick, soggy crust. And one of my most loved breakfasts was a bowl of her warm blackberry soup drizzled with raw honey. Today, my favorite way to eat these plump berries is raw, either layered in a parfait or sprinkled atop a bowl of muesli. Blackberries have a very short season when they are at their sweet, flavorful best. They tend to be mushy, unripe, and exorbitantly priced when available in grocery stores. They are high in fiber and are a good source of vitamin C, antioxidant flavonoids, manganese, and potassium.

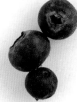

BLUEBERRIES. A superfood if there ever was one, blueberries contain high concentrations of antioxidant and anti-inflammatory compounds such as anthocyanins and proanthocyanidins and are a good source of fiber. The compounds found in blueberries help keep your immune system functioning as it should, help prevent cancer, heart disease, and arthritis, slow down the aging process, act as a laxative, improve sluggish circulation, cleanse the liver and blood, and strengthen cognitive power, to name just a few benefits.

I use fresh and frozen blueberries to make shakes and smoothies and in muesli and parfait recipes, and I use dried blueberries in muesli, confection, and trail mix recipes. Dried blueberries can be quite expensive, but a little does go a long way when you want to add intense blueberry flavor to recipes. Sometimes these little goodies are available only sweetened with apple juice and that's okay. If you have a food dehydrator and access to inexpensive fresh blueberries, making your own dried blueberries is easy and far more cost-effective than purchasing them.

Here in coastal Maine, around about mid-August, the huckleberry, a close cousin of the blueberry, can be enjoyed in the same manner as fresh blueberries.

CANTALOUPES. With their smooth, pale, sunset orange flesh and ambrosia-like fragrance, cantaloupes are wonderfully thirst-quenching and low in calories, a good source of potassium and vitamin C, and extraordinarily high in beta-carotene pigments. I use cantaloupe both fresh and frozen in fruit soups and smoothies. The Crenshaw melon makes a good substitute for cantaloupe when available.

CHERRIES.
Cherries are high in anti-inflammatory, antioxidant, antiaging, and anticancer properties due to a strong presence of flavonoid compounds such as anthocyanin and quercetin, and ellagic acid, another potent antioxidant. In addition to being delicious, cherries are a good source of potassium, magnesium, iron, silicon, vitamin C, and beta-carotene (especially sour cherries), and are a wonderful dietary addition for those suffering from heart disease, arthritis, gout, and various forms of cancer.

Dried cherries add tang to trail mix, muesli, raw candy, and energy bars; fresh cherries are delicious raw during their brief season; and frozen cherries can be added to shakes or smoothies.

CRANBERRIES.
I lived in cranberry country — Cape Cod, Massachusetts — for more than 20 years and have witnessed many cranberry harvests firsthand. What a spectacular sight! Upon flooding the cranberry bog, the buoyant cranberries float to the top, forming a bright burgundy lake. If Mother Nature sets the stage for a picture-postcard-perfect September's day, that lake of cranberry red, being harvested by workers in yellow waders, will visually meld into a crisp, cloudless, brilliant blue autumn sky. Just lovely!

These little fruits are high in antioxidants, antibacterial properties, and flavonoids (especially when raw) and are a good source of vitamin C and fiber. Dried, unsweetened cranberries can be added to trail mix, parfait, muesli, and energy bar recipes. Sometimes they are available sweetened only with apple juice, and that's okay. Occasionally, I make a raw cranberry relish with crushed berries, honey, tangerine peel, and juice — a fresher cousin to cooked cranberry sauce.

CURRANTS. The so-called currants commonly found in the baking or bulk-foods aisle, looking like tiny raisins, aren't really dried currants at all; they are dried black Corinth grapes, sometimes called Zante currants. Who knew? These incorrectly labeled currants are rich in natural sugars, fiber, and antioxidants and are a good source of B vitamins niacin and biotin and calcium, boron, potassium, and iron. Actual currants are difficult to find in domestic markets and tend to be perishable and rather expensive. I use only sweet, chewy dried currants for my trail mix, muesli, parfait, raw candy, and energy bar recipes.

DATES. A most versatile, moist, super-sweet fruit, dates are nature's ready-to-eat raw candy. They are high in calories and natural sugars, fiber, iron, potassium, and phosphorus and are a good fruit source for B vitamins niacin and folic acid. The large, incredibly sweet Medjool dates are my favorites, as I can pit and stuff them with nuts or nut butters and eat only one and call it a complete snack. Smaller, semidry dates, such as the Deglet Noor, are not quite as sweet as the Medjool, nor as moist, but can be used in much the same manner. Dates add sweetness to nut milks and shakes and a cohesive stickiness and sweetness to energy bars and raw candy.

FIGS. There's nothing like a fresh ripe fig. They're a most sensual treat with their heady, sweet aroma, creamy-smooth taste, pinkish red flesh, chubby shape, and tiny nectar-filled seeds that pop and slip between your teeth. While growing up in the southern United States, I had picking access to backyard fig trees and just loved to gorge on the soft, sweet flesh until I was nearly ill. Dried figs, such as the small Black Mission and larger pale, golden brown Turkish or Calimyrna, are readily available and far less expensive than fresh figs. I use them much the same way I do dates, as sweeteners in nut milks and shakes, in energy bars and raw candy, and also in fruit compotes. Dried figs, in particular, rank high in the fiber, natural sugar, calcium, iron, and potassium nutrient categories and provide a nice complement of the B vitamins. They're terrific as a gentle, tasty remedy for constipation.

GRAPEFRUITS. Sweet-tart and ultra-refreshing, grapefruits are rich in potassium, vitamin C, and capillary-strengthening flavonoids and help to stabilize blood sugar. I use grapefruits primarily in fresh-squeezed citrus juice blends or simply enjoy them raw, peeled and sectioned, especially midwinter, when citrus fruits are about the only fresh fruit available up here in Maine.

GRAPES. The seeds and skins of grapes are a potent source of a class of flavonoids called oligomeric proanthocyanidins; put simply, grapes are powerful antioxidants. They act as anti-inflammatories, helping to prevent heart disease and arthritis. Red and purple grapes also contain resveratrol, a compound found in red wine and credited for its health-promoting, life-extending properties that aid in the promotion of cardiovascular health. Grapes are also a decent source of beta-carotene and vitamin C, fiber, phosphorus, and potassium and are quite high in natural sugars. Frozen whole, they taste like tiny bites of grape sorbet and are wonderful eaten on a hot summer's day. They can, of course, also be eaten fresh. (For dried grapes, see entries for Currants and Raisins.)

HONEYDEW MELONS. If available fresh and perfectly ripe from the garden, these juicy melons have a honey-sweet, almost nectarlike flavor. Honeydews have approximately the same nutrients, calories, and thirst-quenching properties as cantaloupes but contain only a minimal amount of beta-carotene. Honeydews are delicious in all the same recipes that feature cantaloupes.

LEMONS. Sour, refreshing, and known for its vitamin C content, lemon juice is beneficial for the health of the liver, gallbladder, and overall digestion. Add fresh-squeezed lemon juice to juice blends or mix it with honey and ginger juice to help heal a sore throat. Stir into a fruit salad and the citric acid in lemons will help prevent the oxidation or browning of apples, pears, and other fruits. Additionally, chewing on a small slice of organic lemon peel makes a great breath freshener!

LIMES. This zippy green citrus fruit is practically identical in nutrient content to lemons. I use limes in fresh-squeezed citrus juice blends and to add a bit of tang to fruit soups.

MANGOES. This luscious, juicy tropical fruit is a terrific source of yellow-orange carotenoid pigments, plus potent enzymes, vitamin C, and potassium, with lesser amounts of vitamin K, calcium, magnesium, and phosphorus. Fresh mangoes are wonderful cut from the pit and eaten plain. Mashed mangoes make a brightly colored, puddinglike layer in parfaits and can be blended in tropical smoothies and added to fruit soups. Unsweetened, unsulfured, dried mango slices are quite leathery and chewy and make a wonderful, colorful addition to trail mix and muesli.

MULBERRIES. I don't often find these tasty berries available fresh, so I use them primarily dried in trail mix and muesli recipes. If you have access to a mulberry tree, try to pick enough of these reddish purple berries to eat fresh and freeze for later. Their dietary contributions are moderate amounts of vitamin C, iron, calcium, and potassium.

NECTARINES. A sweeter, fuzz-free version of the peach, nectarines contribute a moderate amount of several carotenoids and potassium. They are full of exquisite, juicy flavor and make tasty additions to smoothies, shakes, and parfaits when used either fresh or frozen.

ORANGES, TANGELOS, AND TANGERINES. Each of the fruits in this citrus trio contains cancer-fighting phytochemicals and flavonoids, is high in vitamin C, and has moderate amounts of carotenoids, folic acid, potassium, and calcium. My absolute all-time favorite citrus fruit is the Honeybell tangelo, usually available only in February. Nothing beats its sweet, tangy, slightly lime-tinged flavor! I use all of these fruits fresh-squeezed for thirst-quenching juice and in smoothies and shakes.

PAPAYAS. My recipes call for the readily available Hawaiian papaya — about the size of your hand — not the Mexican papaya, which can be the size of a large melon. Papayas are a rich source of the proteolytic enzyme known as papain, which helps to break down or digest protein and may be of aid to those suffering from arthritis by reducing inflammation. Unripe papayas contain more of this enzyme than do ripe ones. They are also high in potassium, fiber, and vitamin C and are a good source of calcium, folate, and carotenoids. Use them fresh in parfait, smoothie, shake, and fruit soup recipes, and enjoy the bright orange, chewy, leathery pieces of unsweetened and unsulfured dried papaya in trail mix and muesli recipes.

PEACHES. These fuzzy cousins of nectarines contain the same basic nutrients, only a bit less of them. I prefer to eat peaches raw when in season, as that is when they are at their juicy best. Fresh or frozen, peaches and nectarines are interchangeable. Use them in smoothies, shakes, and parfaits.

PEARS. The main nutrient contributions from this juicy, fragrant fruit are folic acid, fiber, magnesium, and potassium. If you suffer from constipation, pears can be your best friend, as they add several types of fiber, a mucilaginous consistency, and moisture to the colon. I mainly enjoy pears raw (the big Comice pears being my favorites), cut into slices, and slathered with fresh almond butter. Thick pear nectar is a wonderful addition to cold fruit soups. Dried pears are tasty but tough on the teeth, as they are extremely leathery and chewy — a good hiking food to be savored and eaten slowly.

PERSIMMONS. When I was growing up, my grandfather had a couple of American persimmon trees growing in his northern Georgia pasture. In late fall, after the first frost, these smooth-skinned, hard green fruits, the size of large marbles, would ripen and turn a dusty orange, becoming very soft. The inside of these fruits revealed a few large seeds encased in bright orange flesh and a unique sweet-tart flavor, with an almost slimy-slick, very juicy, mushy consistency. They should be very, very soft with slightly translucent skin before consuming. If you eat them unripe — as I did upon occasion, my impatience getting the best of me — persimmons will instantly produce a peculiar, astringent, fuzzy mouthfeel that is akin to eating a wad of dryer lint.

If you can't find the small American persimmons, you surely will be able to find the larger, baseball-size Japanese varieties in your grocery store. If you have to purchase them slightly unripe and still a bit firm, at least make sure they have a bright orange color. Store them in a paper bag with a banana for up to a week, and they will ripen. The small American persimmons are significantly more nutritious than the Japanese varieties, with plenty of fiber, vitamin C, iron, potassium, and carotenoids. I use persimmons in my Autumn Glow Persimmon Pudding Parfait (page 186) or simply eat them raw.

PINEAPPLES. Pineapples are a rich source of the proteolytic enzyme known as bromelain, which helps to break down or digest protein. Similar to papain, found in papayas, it may reduce inflammation in those suffering from arthritis. The spiky fruits also contribute folic acid, manganese, vitamin C, and potassium. When choosing a pineapple, it should be heavy for its size, "give" slightly to thumb pressure, be golden in color, and smell strongly of sweet pineapple aroma. If you can pull out one of the top leaves with ease, that is another tip-off that it is probably ripe. Enjoy fresh pineapple in smoothies and parfaits and add the chewy, unsweetened, unsulfured, dried pieces to trail mix and muesli recipes.

PRUNES. Dried plums — also known as prunes — have one of the highest levels of antioxidants of all foods available, higher even than blueberries! This means that these little wrinkly brown fruit bites offer a lot of health-promoting, disease-prevention power. Sweet, tasty, chewy prunes are high in natural sugars and a good source of both flavonoids and carotenoids, calcium, potassium, fiber, and iron. And, true to their reputation, they are a gentle remedy for constipation. I like to munch on a few when I have a craving for sweets and also use them in energizing shakes, fruit compotes, and raw candy.

RAISINS. This pantry staple is virtually identical in nutritional content to currants and used in the same types of recipes: trail mix, muesli, parfaits, raw candy, and energy bars. Look for the large black Monukka or Red Flame raisins; both are exceptionally dense, sweet, and chewy.

RASPBERRIES. Deliciously high in fiber, these juicy red berries also provide the B vitamins biotin and niacin, vitamins C and K, manganese, and potassium. Raspberries, like cherries, are also a good source of anti-inflammatory, antioxidant, antiaging, and anticancer properties due to a strong presence of flavonoid anthocyanin compounds and ellagic acid. I feast on in-season raspberries purchased from a farm stand or picked from wild-growing canes. Fresh or frozen, they're terrific in smoothie, shake, parfait, and fruit soup recipes or sprinkled atop a bowl of muesli. Dried raspberries can be difficult to find and expensive at times and are frequently treated with sulfur to preserve their bright red color. If available unsulfured, they make sweet-tart, chewy additions to trail mix recipes. Making dried raspberries is a cost-effective option if you happen to own a food dehydrator and are near a source of fresh, inexpensive garden, farm-grown, or wild berries.

STRAWBERRIES. Sweet, red, juicy locally grown strawberries — my favorite kind — are high in vitamin C, folic acid, and potassium, and, like raspberries, they are a good source of flavonoid anthocyanin compounds and ellagic acid. Fresh or frozen, they are tasty in smoothies, shakes, and parfaits or sliced atop muesli. Like raspberries, dried strawberries can be difficult to find at times and expensive and are frequently treated with sulfur to preserve their bright red color. If available unsulfured, they make sweet additions to trail mixes. You can always dehydrate and preserve your own, if you have a food dehydrator and live near a pick-your-own farm or can harvest them from your garden or growing wild.

WATERMELON. This thirst-quenching fruit is loaded with natural sugars, carotenoids such as lycopene and beta-carotene, and potassium.

If you're feeling bloated, drinking several large glasses of watermelon juice will act as a natural diuretic and dramatically reduce that waterlogged feeling, as will making a strong tea from the raw, cracked seeds and consuming several glasses. I eat watermelon raw and also as a refreshing juice with a few mint leaves tossed in for zing.

Vegetables

Colorful, versatile, tasty, low in both sugar and calories, and chock-full of vitamins, minerals, and fiber, vegetables are nature's good-for-you energy foods. There are no bad vegetables, and you can never eat too many; if only this could be said for all foods! The best vegetables are available in-season and locally from farmers' markets and co-ops. Try to buy organic when available.

Raw Food Storage

Paradoxically, the warmth, light, and air which impart the "living forces" to growing foods will destroy them after they have been harvested. Take hay, for example, which is livestock's chief source of complete vitamins. A farmer will store his hay, protecting it as much as possible from light, heat, and moving air currents. Years ago there were dairies which bottled milk in amber-colored bottles to protect the milk from light. The milk was to be kept refrigerated and sealed except when poured for use. The same principles apply to all "living food," once harvested. The food should be protected as much as possible from warmth, light, and air.

— Ann Wigmore, *Recipes for Longer Life*

AVOCADOS. Although avocados are technically a fruit, most people think of them as a vegetable. They are full of fat, but it's healthful fat, primarily monounsaturated, the same type you would find in olive oil and macadamia nuts. Avocados are quite filling and fiber-filled, with plenty of beta-carotene and lutein — the "eye-health" antioxidant. They are an excellent source of potassium and a good source of the B vitamins, especially niacin and folic acid, with lesser quantities of easily absorbed vitamin E, iron, copper, magnesium, and calcium. I adore them raw with a simple sprinkling of sea salt. I also use avocados in creamy, raw vegetable soups and dips. The smaller, rougher-textured, bumpy-skinned Hass avocados are sweet, creamy, and preferable to the Florida avocados, which have smooth skin and a more chunky, watery consistency.

BELL PEPPERS. The bell pepper, sometimes called a sweet pepper, is green when immature, but as it ripens turns red, yellow, orange, or purple, depending upon the variety. The brighter the color, the sweeter the flavor. Nutritionally, bell peppers are rich in vitamin C and loaded with red or yellow carotenoid pigments. They're a pretty good source of potassium, folic acid, and fiber, too. Fresh bell peppers are a key ingredient in gazpacho soup and vegetable juice blends.

CARROTS. This crunchy orange "rabbit food" is rich in carotenoids, the antioxidant compounds that boost every aspect of vigorous health. They are also a good source of calcium, potassium, and fiber, with lesser amounts of vitamins C and B, magnesium, phosphorus, and selenium. I enjoy drinking carrot juice alone (a veritable health-food meal in a glass) or in vegetable juice blends. The juice also makes a terrific raw-soup ingredient. Carrot sticks are quite tasty when dipped in raw almond butter or sesame tahini and eaten as a quick, highly nutritious snack.

CELERY. Nutritionally speaking, celery is a good source of folic acid, sodium, and potassium and a rich source of silicon, important for the health of your bones and connective tissue. Celery adds a touch of salty flavor to vegetable juice blends and a bit of crunch to gazpacho soup, and when cut into sticks can be stuffed with nut butter and eaten as a quick snack.

CUCUMBERS. This cooling, light crunchy vegetable can quench your thirst with its high water content. When eaten with the peel, cucumbers contain moderate amounts of silicon, chlorophyll, potassium, folic acid, and vitamin C. I use cucumbers in vegetable juice blends and soup recipes. There's nothing quite as refreshing as a chilled cuke — fresh from the garden and sprinkled with sea salt — on a hot summer's day.

GARLIC. Garlic is one of the most revered immune-system-boosting, antibacterial, antiviral, and antifungal foods on the planet and is often eaten roasted as a vegetable, added to stews and sauces for its robust flavor, and sliced raw as a salad and dressing ingredient. In my *Raw Energy* recipes, I use it primarily as a powerful, pungent, circulation-stimulating seasoning in raw vegetable soups and dips. If you're a true garlic aficionado, then by all means feel free to use a heavier hand with the garlic in my recipes, but if garlic tends to wreak havoc with your digestive system, as it does mine, then use only the recommended amounts.

JALAPEÑO PEPPERS. Small, hot, jalapeño peppers are similar in nutrient content to bell peppers. They derive their heat from capsaicin, a vasodilator that produces warmth when applied to the skin and, when consumed, increases circulation and metabolism. Spicy jalapeños add bite to vegetable juice blends and dip recipes. Raw jalapeño peppers are also wonderful stuffed with vegetable pâté or spread and eaten as vegetarian "poppers."

ONIONS. A member of the Allium family — as are leeks, garlic, chives, and scallions — onions contain strong sulfuric compounds that are necessary for the health of hair, skin, nails, and digestive tract. They also contribute folic acid, calcium, vitamin C, and potassium. I use finely minced onions in raw gazpacho soup and vegetable dips, pâtés, and spreads.

POTATOES, WHITE AND SWEET. Soon after I moved to Maine, new friends who just happened to be potato farmers, among other professions, introduced me to an exciting new taste sensation: freshly dug, *raw* Kennebec white potatoes sprinkled with sea salt and vinegar. "Yuck!"

you say? Don't knock it till you try it! When ultra fresh, the taste and texture are similar to that of a jicama — crispy but a little less sweet. White potatoes are a good source of potassium and vitamins C and B. Their orange-fleshed cousins, sweet potatoes, are very rich in orange-yellow carotene pigments and a good source of potassium. My main use for potatoes is to thinly slice, coat with olive oil, and dehydrate them, creating healthful "potato chips," avoiding the trans fat found in many fried chips and preserving the whole potato flavor. When dehydrated, they yield crispy, slightly chewy treats. You can partake of them plain, salted, or with vegetable dips and pâtés.

SCALLIONS. These long green members of the Onion family are a good source of folic acid, beta-carotene, vitamin C, sulfur compounds, and potassium. I use them as I do chives, finely chopped and stirred into vegetable dip and pâté recipes. Scallions contribute a wonderful spark of bright green color and oniony flavor.

SPINACH. Want to be strong, energetic, and healthy like Popeye? Then eat your spinach. It's one of the vegetable all-stars as far as I'm concerned. Spinach is loaded with antioxidants such as lutein, beta-carotene, several anti-inflammatory flavonoids, vitamins C and K, folic acid, iron, calcium, potassium, and magnesium. I mainly enjoy it in salads, drizzled with balsamic vinegar, or minced and added to vegetable dip recipes.

SUMMER SQUASHES, YELLOW AND GREEN.

Nutritionally speaking, these common summer squashes make quite a good contribution of potassium, folic acid, and antioxidants beta-carotene and lutein to the diet. When enhanced with tasty seasonings, they make wonderful additions to dips, raw soups, and hummus recipes. If you're a gardener and happen to have a few large yellow or zucchini squashes on hand in mid-summer (and who doesn't?), they can be sliced and used to make delicious dehydrated vegetable chips.

TOMATOES.

Vine-ripened tomatoes, picked at the height of their summer flavor, offer thirst-quenching, spectacularly sweet taste sensations that can be relished in chilled summer soups and vegetable juice blends. I often eat tomatoes raw with a sprinkling of sea salt and fresh, chopped basil leaves, or, if I have a particularly bountiful harvest, will slice and dehydrate them to add to recipes all winter long. Freezing raw tomato juice is a great way to add summer freshness to winter soups. If superior taste, texture, and freshness aren't reasons enough to grow your own tomatoes, did you know that vine-ripened tomatoes have twice the amount of vitamin C than those grown in a hothouse or those that are picked green and artificially ripened with ethylene gas (as are most supermarket tomatoes)? They are also higher in natural sugars, potassium, and lutein and lycopene — carotenoids that, respectively, promote eye health and protect against several types of cancer.

Oils

All oils, whether derived from nuts, seeds, vegetables, or fruits, are basically pure fat. If properly extracted without the use of chemicals, excessive heat, or processing, they are very tasty, revealing unique flavor dimensions of any foods they accompany. The following oils are quite good for you, being rich in essential fatty acids and other nutrients that your body needs to maintain energy and health. They are also calorically dense, with 1 tablespoon yielding approximately 12 to 14 grams of fat and 120 calories, so use them judiciously in your daily diet.

COCONUT OIL. Ahhh . . . the warm tropical fragrance and taste of raw, organic, unrefined, cold-pressed, extra-virgin coconut oil. If you love coconut, you can even slather this rich oil on your skin and hair as a moisturizing treatment. Coconut oil, sometimes referred to as coconut butter because it becomes solid at room temperature, is one of the healthiest fats you can ingest. Though it is primarily a saturated fat (which is fine, especially if eaten raw), it contains medium-chain good fats with approximately 50 percent of a particularly important fatty acid known as lauric acid, which supports the metabolism and has potent antiviral, antibacterial, and immune-enhancing properties. I like to add aromatic, flavorful coconut oil to smoothie, shake, and confection recipes. It also comes in handy to grease hands and pans when working with sticky dough.

FLAXSEED OIL. I love the taste, texture, and color of flaxseed oil — slightly nutty, rich, thick, smooth, and dark golden brown in color. Look for organically produced, unrefined, cold-pressed oil with lignans (phytonutrients with a protective effective against cancer). The bottle should be made of dark glass or plastic and located in the refrigerated section, as this oil is highly perishable. Always check the pressing date and expiration date on the label to make sure it's fresh. Flaxseed oil typically contains 45 to 65 percent alpha-linolenic acid or omega-3 fatty acid and is one of the best vegetarian sources for this nutrient, which acts as an anti-inflammatory agent, protecting against such conditions as arthritis, colitis, cardiovascular disease, PMS, cancer, psoriasis, and acne roseacea, among others. I use flaxseed oil, or a combination of flax and extra-virgin olive oil, to lend a hearty rich flavor to homemade salad dressing.

OLIVE OIL. When shopping for a top-quality, nutritionally superior olive oil, seek out organically produced, unrefined, extra-virgin oil from the first stone-crushed cold pressing and look for a harvesting and bottling date on the label. This thick green oil contains potent antioxidant compounds, plentiful enzymes, and a high percentage of monounsaturated fat, which is extremely heart-healthy. It's a great lubricant for your internal organs and a moisturizing agent when applied to your skin and hair. In this book, I use it when making trail mix, pesto, and dehydrated vegetable chips.

Salty Condiments

I can pass up a rich, gooey dessert any time, but offer me a handful (or bowlful) of crunchy, salty pecans or dehydrated potato chips, and I'm in heaven. I have a "salt-fat tooth," as do many Americans, that, once excited, can be hard to tame. The salty flavors I use in the *Raw Energy* recipes are derived from two fairly healthful sources, unrefined sea salt and raw soy sauce, and I use both judiciously, as flavor intensifiers or enhancers. Remember, a little salt goes a long way.

SEA SALT. Most Americans crave the taste of salt, eat far too much of it, and use the wrong kind at that. The familiar iodized table salt — cheaply sold in the grocery store and included in just about every convenience food available — has been processed at very high temperatures, bleached, and demineralized and includes added anticaking chemicals to keep it "free-flowing." It acts in the body as a poison rather than the necessary nutrient it can be. Sea salt, Celtic Sea Salt brand in particular, on the other hand, is hand-harvested from one of the most pristine coastal regions of France, then sun- and wind-dried. It retains a slight bit of moisture and grayish ocean-water color, and contains a natural balance of minerals and trace elements that are beneficial to most diets. This type of salt has an appealing texture and is delicious when sprinkled on fresh vegetables, mango, papaya, and avocado slices and is used in many of the recipes throughout this book.

SOY SAUCE. If you enjoy the rich, salty taste of soy sauce, there are two varieties of raw, unpasteurized, enzyme-packed soy sauces that I recommend; one is Bragg Liquid Aminos, made from aged soy-beans and water, and the other is Nama Shoyu, which is made from aged soybeans, wheat, and water. Soy sauce adds a savory flavor to trail mix, vegetable chips, and vegetable soups.

Herbs and Spices: Fresh and Dried

For thousands of years, herbs and spices have been used to transform bland, common foods and dishes into extraordinary gustatory delights. Their flavors run the gamut from subtle and sublime, to sweet and savory, to fiery and pungent, depending upon the amounts used and the particular herbs or spices chosen. Though not generally eaten in quantity, they do add beneficial trace amounts of vitamins and minerals to the diet, so quality and freshness are very important. In addition to individual herbs, I use various traditional herb and spice blends in some of my recipes to enhance flavor, such as chili powder, Italian seasoning, all-purpose seasoning, curry powder, and lemon-pepper seasoning.

Purchase only organically grown fresh and dried herbs and try to grow as many fresh herbs as you can in your garden or in pots. Many, if not most, imported dried herbs and spices are grown with herbicides and pesticides and often irradiated or treated with ozone, sulfur gas, or other chemicals when they enter this country. Avoid these whenever possible. Contact the grower, manufacturer, distributor, or store manager and ask questions about the origins and processing of the products you are purchasing. See the Resources section (page 264) for a listing of companies that offer organically grown herbs and spices of unsurpassed quality, depth, taste, color, and aroma.

BASIL. A green, slightly sweet, pungent, mildly peppery member of the Mint family that, when fresh and in season, causes pesto fans to swoon with anticipation of tasting that rich, oily, succulent, tangy spread that is deliciously up to the challenge of topping almost any food of grain or vegetable origin. Can you tell that I simply adore basil? In addition to using fresh-picked basil in my pesto recipe, I also use jumbo "lettuce leaf" basil leaves like tortillas and wrap them around thick slices of tomatoes or stuff them with vegetable spread.

CAYENNE. This pepper's color is vibrant and electric, flavor is pungently hot, and sensation is one of a burning nature if you get the powder in your nose or eyes. I use a mere smidgen of cayenne pepper to add spicy heat and circulatory stimulation to the occasional fruit juice, energy bar, raw candy, trail mix, and vegetable dip recipe. It also pairs deliciously with raw cocoa.

CHIVES. Often confused with scallions, chives are a member of the onion family, and are a good source of beta-carotene, vitamin C, folic acid, calcium, iron, potassium, and sulfur compounds. When the green tubular tops are finely chopped and stirred into vegetable dip and pâté recipes, chives contribute a wonderful spark of bright green color and mild, onionlike flavor.

CINNAMON. A wonderful digestive aid, cinnamon has a comforting, warming, sweet, pungent, and slightly acidic flavor that most of us associate with grandma's kitchen, apple pie, hot apple cider, and cinnamon buns. Ground cinnamon is made from the powdered inner bark of the cinnamon tree. I use it in smoothie, shake, energy bar, trail mix, muesli, parfait, and raw candy recipes — almost everything!

GINGERROOT. Fresh, delicious, warming, and zippy, ginger is a remarkable healing spice to consume when you have a sore throat or a head or chest cold, suffer from indigestion, or need waking up in the morning. I use zingy, stimulating gingerroot processed in several ways: juiced, finely minced, or thinly sliced when making juice blends or my Morning Power Shot recipe (page 127). Occasionally, I'll use crystallized ginger in energy bar, trail mix, and raw candy recipes.

MINT. One of my former herb teachers, Rosemary Gladstar, calls mint "a blast of pure green energy." Right she is! Crush a fresh mint leaf between your fingers and take a deep whiff; the sharp, cooling aroma acts as an uplifting tonic for the emotions and the senses. Simply sipping a cup of pleasantly flavored mint tea stimulates the circulation, refreshes, and invigorates the body. I add fresh mint leaves to energizing juice blends and as an edible garnish to raw fruit soups.

NUTMEG. This wintery spice is derived from the ground seed of the evergreen nutmeg tree. Its sweet, warm, piquant, slightly bitter flavor is delicately nutty, and subtlety reminiscent of pine or evergreen with a dash of citrus. Even though its aroma seems rather modest, nutmeg is deceptively intense and can easily overpower other flavors, so use sparingly. I enjoy its full-bodied taste in shake, energy bar, trail mix, and raw candy recipes.

PARSLEY. Not merely a plate garnish to be tossed aside like so much leftover food, parsley, whether Italian flat-leaf or the common curly variety, is quite high in blood-building chlorophyll and iron, antioxidant carotenoids lutein and zeaxanthin for eye health, beta-carotene, plus vitamin K, calcium, potassium, and flavonoids. Last but not least, it's a fabulous breath freshener. I love the aromatic, green, slightly tangy, peppery flavor it lends to raw vegetable soups, dips, and juices.

Parsley, Nature's Blood Builder

Dark green leafy vegetables — parsley, spinach, watercress, and many others — are rich in chlorophyll, the green pigment that most plants require for photosynthesis. It is sometimes called "the blood of the plant" in that it is chemically nearly identical to human hemoglobin. Chlorophyll stimulates red blood cell production. Additionally, dark green leafy vegetables contain many nutrients, including vitamin K and iron, which are necessary for building healthy blood.

PEPPER. Derived from the dried, unripe berry of the tropical, vining pepper shrub, black pepper has a sharp flavor that adds an invigorating edge to many foods. I'm a big fan of all things peppery and like to add it to vegetable dip, chip, spread, and raw vegetable soup recipes.

Specialty Ingredients

These ingredients don't seem to fit into a particular type of food category, but each has something distinctive to offer your raw snack recipes — a unique flavor, nutritive quality, unusual texture, or all three — and each is wonderfully good for you. I recommend that you give them all a try, at least once, and see which ones entice you the most.

BEE POLLEN. These tiny, honey-flavored, powdery-textured golden nuggets are formed when honeybees combine with nectar millions of microscopic pollen grains collected from flowers. Bee pollen is a rich source of amino acids, live enzymes, and most B vitamins, including folic acid, and almost every other essential nutrient we need to survive and thrive. It is classified by some nutritionists as a true, complete superfood, strength builder, and brain food. I add it to shake and energy bar recipes to enhance stamina and rebuild long-term deficient *chi* (energy), but my favorite way to consume this wonder food is to simply eat 2 teaspoons daily — straight from the jar. Yummy! If you are prone to grass or flower pollen allergies, try to buy only locally produced bee pollen, as regular consumption of small amounts can, in many cases, help temper your allergic reaction to these particular plants.

BARLEY GRASS POWDER. This alkalizing cereal grass is high in enzymes and blood-building chlorophyll and loaded with trace amounts of vitamins and minerals. It's quite calming and healing for an irritated digestive tract and a great alternative for those who don't tolerate wheatgrass well. Use it as an energizing, pick-me-up additive to fresh juices.

CAROB POWDER. Also known as St. John's bread, carob is a brown, pod-shaped fruit from an evergreen tree widely cultivated in the Mediterranean. The powder is derived from the dried, sweet pulp and is often referred to as a healthful "chocolate alternative" mainly because it has a somewhat similar taste and texture as cocoa powder but is missing the caffeine and other stimulating chemicals contained in cocoa. Carob powder is most commonly available roasted but can also be purchased raw. It is a good source of B vitamins, calcium, iron, potassium, and pectin. I use it in the same types of recipes as I do raw cocoa powder, below.

COCOA POWDER. Raw cocoa powder? Yes! Nearly all of the cocoa powder on the market is the end result of the multi-step processing needed to create chocolate liquor, which involves cleaning, fermenting, sorting, roasting, cracking, and grinding of the cacao seed or cocoa bean. But now there is actually raw cocoa powder (also called cacao powder) available, made without all that heat. It is dark, rich, bitter, quite high in health- and beauty-boosting antioxidant flavonoids, calcium, magnesium, manganese, sulfur, potassium, phosphorus, zinc, iron, copper, protein, healthful fat, and fiber, and sinfully delicious! I'm a chocoholic — I admit it — and I like to add raw cocoa powder's chocolaty goodness to almond milk, shake, raw candy, and energy bar recipes. Mixed with honey or agave nectar, it even makes a fabulous raw chocolate syrup!

CACAO NIBS. These dark, roughly textured bits are the raw version of chocolate chips, without all the sugar and additives, and can be added to any recipe where you want a crunchy, bitter chocolate flavor. Finely ground cacao nibs become raw cacao powder.

FLAVORINGS. I sometimes like to use vanilla, orange, peppermint, and almond flavorings to enhance the taste of smoothies and shakes. It takes only a small amount, ¼ to ½ teaspoon, to alter the flavor of a particular recipe, so don't get too heavy-handed. Oil-based, glycerin-based, or alcohol-based formulations are available, but none of these is 100 percent raw. Please follow your particular brand's label directions for use in these recipes.

SIBERIAN GINSENG. Ginseng root is imbued with almost magical qualities. Also called *eleuthero,* Siberian ginseng has similar properties and health benefits to Chinese, or *panax,* ginseng. Best known for improving stamina and endurance and boosting circulation, it should be taken consistently over a period of time, as it helps restore vitality deep within the tissues, thereby increasing resistance to disease. It is also believed to bestow wisdom and promote longevity upon the consumer. A powerful, potent plant! I mix the bland-tasting powdered root into energy ball and occasionally raw candy recipes and try to consume one or two of these fortifying sweet treats every day to help maintain my get-up-and-go.

SPIRULINA POWDER. This blue-green micro-algae, grown in fresh water, is high in vegetable protein, antioxidant carotenoids, blood-building chlorophyll and iron, essential fatty acids, and many other vitamins and minerals. Powdered spirulina, though quite nutritious, tastes akin to seaweed — a bit fishy — and is best disguised in heavily flavored shake, smoothie, and energy bar recipes.

VINEGAR, APPLE CIDER. Always purchase raw apple cider vinegar. Unless it says "raw" on the label, it has been heated to high temperatures and filtered, and the beneficial enzymes destroyed. I prefer Bragg Organic Apple Cider Vinegar. It is raw, unfiltered, loaded with live enzymes and potassium, tastes deliciously sweet-tart and tangy, and has a rich, brownish color. This brand of raw vinegar is made from fresh crushed apples that are aged and allowed to ferment in wooden barrels until ripe and ready to be bottled. Blend it with either flaxseed or olive oil, various herbs such as oregano, basil, marjoram, rosemary, and thyme, garlic, onions, black pepper, and sea salt to create one of the best raw salad dressings you'll ever taste.

WHEATGRASS POWDER. The nutrient properties and uses of wheatgrass are virtually the same as barley grass powder, discussed above, but wheatgrass tends to taste a touch sweeter.

Kitchen Equipment Essentials

Making raw snack goodies requires minimal equipment, compared with what you need to make baked, roasted, fried, sautéed, toasted, grilled, broiled, or boiled food. With a couple of good sharp knives, a food processor, mesh strainer, cutting board, medium-size bowl and spoon, set of measuring cups, and a blender, you can create more than three-quarters of the recipes in this book. If you don't happen to have access to every piece of equipment or gadget listed below, don't let that stop you from snacking on raw goodness. Once you begin to enjoy raw snacking on a regular basis using the tools you already have, and realize how yummy and health-building the recipes are, then you may want to invest in the nice-to-haves such as a mandoline or spiral slicer, or in the more expensive tools, such as a quality juicer and food dehydrator, or perhaps even upgrade the equipment you currently own to fancier gizmos that offer more options.

Outfit your kitchen with the right tools for the job and you will arrive at your desired recipe destination faster, with flair and with pleasurable ease. Making raw snacks is supposed to be *fun,* not daunting, so enjoy the ride!

BLENDER. My blender is one of my most frequently used tools for making raw snacks. When purchasing a blender, be sure to buy one with a strong motor, preferably one that can grind ice cubes into a fine crystal "snow cone" consistency. A blender can be used for making frosty shakes and slushes with frozen and softened dried fruit; blending smoothies, frozen fruit creams, and puddings; grinding soaked and softened nuts into nut milk or soft cashew butter; puréeing fruit or vegetable soups; and blending vegetable dips, pâtés, and spreads.

BOWLS. I prefer to use bowls of melamine, wood composite, stainless steel, glass, pottery, and the newer flexible silicone (this one's really handy). Avoid using aluminum and copper bowls when blending acid-based foods such as chopped tomatoes, citrus fruits, and vinegar dressings, as these metals can leach out into your recipe and discolor your food.

CITRUS REAMER. I use an old-fashioned glass reamer for extracting small quantities of juice (1 cup or less) from lemons, limes, oranges, tangelos, tangerines, and very small grapefruits.

COFFEE OR SPICE GRINDER. This small appliance is convenient, inexpensive, and powerful; perfect for grinding small batches of nuts, seeds, or whole small spices (not whole nutmeg, though) when a blender or food processor would be much too large. Keep a separate grinder for your coffee beans, or everything else will taste and smell like coffee!

CUTTING BOARD. Plastic, wood, or bamboo, the choice is up to you; just make sure to keep it scrupulously clean at all times. I rely on a thick wooden cutting board and frequently place one of those flexible plastic cutting sheets on top. The thin plastic folds or bends, and enables you to conveniently transfer your chopped ingredient to the blender, food processor, or juicer without spilling a single piece. No scraping required!

DEHYDRATOR. A dehydrator is not a lightweight conventional oven, but it could be considered a "raw food oven." Instead of baking, broiling, or roasting foods at high temperatures, it gently evaporates moisture from food using a warm air current that surrounds the food but doesn't cook it, thus preserving the food's enzymes. Sliced fruits, vegetables, soaked nuts, and prepared raw recipes such as energy bars and cookies take on a heartier, denser, firmer, sometimes crispier texture with a richer, more concentrated flavor when dehydrated.

Many dehydrators will allow you to dry food at temperatures ranging from 85°F to 150°F (29–66°C). I never dehydrate any higher than 115°F (46°C), lest the food's enzymes be destroyed. I use and recommend the Excalibur brand of dehydrator, as I feel it does a very effective job, but there are other brands on the market. Do a little research prior to purchasing. Whichever brand you choose, be sure to follow the manufacturer's instructions for general use, maintenance, and food placement, but follow my particular recipe instructions for temperature setting and duration of drying time.

FOOD PROCESSOR. This piece of equipment is a kitchen must-have for making raw snacks. Don't buy a cheap one, as their motors tend to burn out quickly; a quality, middle-of-the road brand should serve quite nicely. A food processor will quickly shred, slice, chop, mince, purée, or grind nearly any type of ingredient. The "S" blade allows you create dip, spread, and pâté recipes with ease and grind dough for energy bar and raw confection recipes. The slicing disk is useful for producing large quantities of evenly cut slices of potatoes or vegetables for vegetable chips.

FILE GRATER. This handheld tool, commonly known by the brand name Microplane, is used for removing the zest from citrus rinds and grating fresh ginger and nutmeg.

FOOD CHOPPER. This popular kitchen tool is handier than pulling out the blender or food processor when you need to chop less than 2 cups of an ingredient. As you pump the handle up and down, the small, durable, stainless steel rotating blades uniformly chop small amounts of vegetables, hard fruits, or nuts in the attached container in mere seconds.

GARLIC PRESS. If you're a garlic lover, then a garlic press is essential kitchen gadgetry. I prefer the heavy-duty metal presses that can really stand up to pressure. Avoid the ultra-cheap plastic kinds, as they have a tendency to break or snap apart. Whatever kind you choose, make sure it's easy to clean.

JUICER. An electric citrus juicer is handy when I yearn for a big, quick glass of fresh orange, grapefruit, or Honeybell tangelo juice or when I want to make a juice blend or smoothie and need to extract more than 1 cup of citrus juice. I also have a large fruit and vegetable extractor that produces fresh juice with a minimum amount of heat and friction. I like the Green Star brand; it crushes, grinds, and compresses the foods rather than simply grating them at high speeds, as other juicers do, so that you receive the maximum amount of nutrients possible and a drier residual pulp. Granted, it is an expensive, heavy machine, costing several hundred dollars, but I feel that it's worth every penny. There are many different brands and types of juicers on the market, ranging in price from approximately $100 to nearly $1,000. It is not necessary to have a juicer, but it is a wonderful tool for adding the freshest raw juices to your diet. I urge you to buy the highest quality that you can afford and do some homework before purchasing.

KNIVES. Any chef will tell you that a sharp knife is a safer, more effective knife. If you don't already own a set of quality knives, then please make the investment. Also, purchase a knife block or storage case for your knives and a quality sharpening tool.

MANDOLINE. This time-saving, cleverly designed, manual kitchen tool enables you to make short work of processing a pile of vegetables that needs to be uniformly-sized slices or julienne. I use a mandoline for slicing potatoes, summer and winter squashes, and jicamas when I want to make dehydrated vegetable chip recipes. This can be a rather dangerous piece of equipment due to its exposed razor-sharp blades, so please keep out of the hands of children and don't use if your own hands are not steady — fingers and knuckles can be severely cut! Always use the protective equipment that comes with your mandoline. Also, avoid purchasing cheap, flexible, flimsy, plastic models and opt for either thicker, heavier, sturdier plastic or a more expensive, stainless steel French model.

NUT MILK BAG. This fine-mesh or linen bag (mine is approximately 8 inches wide by 10 inches long) is specially made for straining the pulp, skins, and any sweetening fruit bits from freshly ground nut milk. You can also use a sprouting bag.

SPIRAL SLICER. Also referred to as a spiralizer, this nifty, inexpensive gadget is not necessary but is fun to have! It enables you to create a variety of neat shapes with vegetables: flat or ruffled spirals, slices, and thin vegetable "spaghetti" strands. Kids love it! Try your hand at making fresh raw zucchini "spaghetti" and topping it with raw pesto . . . out of this world! It's also a great gadget for quickly making evenly thin slices of white or sweet potatoes.

STORAGE CONTAINERS. I use all kinds of storage containers, depending upon the particular type of food or recipe, length of storage time, and where the food will be stored: dark cabinet, refrigerator, or freezer.

Glass jars are good for storing nuts, seeds, grains, dried herbs, muesli, and other dry ingredients in the cupboard and also finished products such as trail mix. Glass jars can easily be decorated with customized labels, twine, ribbon, and fabric and used as gift containers as well.

Plastic tubs are good for storing dough that you want to chill overnight, for soaking nuts and seeds, and for storing prepared foods such as trail mix, energy bars, and raw confections.

I like to use ziplock freezer bags to store raw ingredients such as nuts, seeds, and grains in the freezer or refrigerator — also perfect for storing trail mix and muesli.

Decorative tins make wonderful presentation packages for sharing your raw snacks as gifts during times of celebration. Line them with tissue paper, plastic wrap, or waxed paper and place your raw confection, trail mix, or energy bar goodies inside and you have a gorgeous gift, all set for healthful festive noshing.

VEGETABLE PEELER. To be honest, I don't often use a peeler. I simply scrub my fruits and vegetables prior to use with a rough scrubby sponge or vegetable brush and leave the skin intact. If I do need to remove the wax coating from foods such as cucumbers or apples, I actually prefer the control I get with a small, very sharp paring knife. You decide.

Chapter 3
RAW SNACK PREP 101: LEARNING HOW TO "UNCOOK"

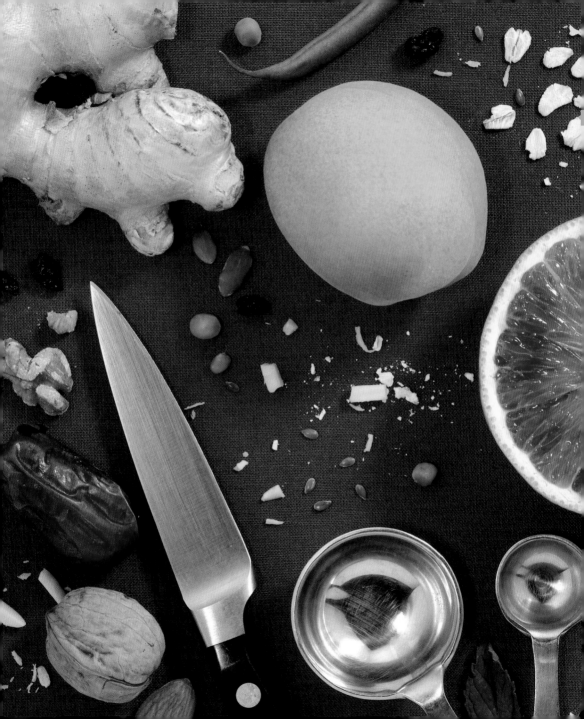

*N*ever fear — no great culinary prowess is necessary to make my delicious raw snacks. Your basic kitchen skills, sometimes applied in unusual ways, will see you through these recipes. In the kitchen, I believe in keeping all things as simple as possible — from ingredient preparation to cleanup. Making raw snacks couldn't be simpler or more enjoyable.

Dehydrating

As explained in the Equipment section (page 81), a dehydrator can be thought of as a very low-temperature "raw food oven." Each recipe that requires the use of a dehydrator will instruct you as to how to prepare the food and load the dehydrator. Due to several factors, such as humidity levels, degree of moisture in the foods, the number of total foods in the dehydrator, and thickness of the foods you are drying, dehydrating times will vary. The more moisture in the air and in the food, the longer it takes to achieve the end result. The suggested dehydrating times given in the recipes are merely guidelines, so you may want to check the progress of your food or recipe every few hours or so, especially if you are new to using the machine, until you get a feel for how long things take to complete. Remember, too, that not all brands of dehydrators have the same rate of flow or degree of warm air circulation.

Soaking Nuts and Seeds

When a recipe calls for raw nuts and seeds, most often the familiar crunchy, dry texture is desired, such as when making many of my trail mix and raw confection recipes. But there are a few recipes that call for soaking and softening nuts and seeds in water, such as when making almond or walnut milk or vegetable dips and spreads that call for a seed or nut paste base.

Nuts and seeds contain enzyme inhibitors in their skins — a natural protective factor that allows nuts, seeds, and beans to remain dormant until soaked with water (most often in the form of rain), preparing them to sprout and grow into a plant. This chemical in their skins is slightly bitter-tasting and can interfere with digestibility. Soaking reduces the enzyme inhibitors in the skin and increases enzyme availability, making soaked nuts and seeds easier to digest. Soaking first and then dehydrating nuts and seeds is a good way to duplicate that delicious, crunchy "roasted" flavor and texture without the use of high heat. I use this method on occasion, when making some trail mix recipes.

To soak, place dry nuts or seeds in a large bowl, covered with an inch or two of purified water — enough water so that the nuts or seeds can easily swim around. Place the bowl on a stable surface and cover with

An Additive to Watch Out For

Keep an eye out for that nasty chemical MSG (monosodium glutamate), a neurotropic drug (a substance that affects the nervous system) used by food manufacturers the world over to "enhance" the taste of food. It doesn't actually improve flavors so much as hide the taste of staleness, sourness, and bitterness. If you've eaten in a Chinese restaurant, you've no doubt experienced the side effects of MSG: lightheadedness, tingling, bloating, fatigue, nausea, blurred vision, shortness of breath, flushing — to name just a few. MSG lurks in varying amounts in ingredients such as autolyzed yeast, texturized vegetable protein, natural flavorings, sodium caseinate, calcium caseinate, hydrolyzed protein, hydrolyzed vegetable protein, and yeast extract. Dough conditioner, an ingredient in many commercial breads, is an MSG-like ingredient and should also be avoided.

a paper towel or porous cloth to keep out any bugs or floating dust and debris. Your nuts or seeds will swell in size and absorb some of the water. Drain and rinse the nuts or seeds at the end of the allotted soaking time. This draining and rinsing process removes acidity and enzyme inhibitors. Do not use the soaking water in any recipe. The specific amount of time necessary to soak nuts or seeds will be indicated in the particular recipe and can range from 2 hours to overnight. Generally, the harder the nut, the longer the soaking time.

Soaking Dried Fruit

Recipes that include dried fruit will specify whether the fruit is to be soaked or used as is, in its dried state. I soak dried fruits to soften and rehydrate tough or leathery ones when making fruit compote, raw jam, or marmalade, or when I want to easily blend them with other ingredients into smoothies or shakes. Soaking dried fruits is done the same way as soaking nuts and seeds, described above, except that you don't need to rinse at the end of the soaking time, as there are no enzyme inhibitors or bitter taste to eliminate. You can chill and drink the soak water if you wish, or add it to a smoothie; it's especially sweet and thirst-quenching. The amount of time necessary to soak fruits will be indicated in the particular recipe and can range from 2 hours to overnight.

Plumped fruits such as prunes or apricots can be delectably seasoned with cinnamon or nutmeg and eaten with a spoon and enjoyed as a sweet, energizing breakfast or snack, alone, or atop a bowl of muesli.

Soaking Oats

Soaking raw, flaked, or whole oat groats tenderizes their dry texture and allows their smooth, mild flavor to develop a bit of creamy richness. Soaked oats are used mainly when preparing raw cereal, such as muesli, and parfait recipes.

To soak oat groats, simply place the amount needed in a large bowl and cover with 2 inches of water. Place the bowl on a stable surface and cover with a paper towel or porous cloth to keep out any bugs, floating dust, or debris. Your groats will swell in size and absorb a good bit of the soak water, so be sure always to use purified or distilled water. Drain and rinse the groats at the end of the allotted soaking time. Do not use the soak water in any recipe, as it may taste bitter. The specific amount of time necessary to soak oat groats will be indicated in the particular recipe, but I generally allow them to soak and soften overnight.

Unlike the tougher oat groats, oat flakes, or rolled oats, do not need to be soaked in water first. Muesli and parfait recipes that contain dry oat flakes will call for some type of nut milk or fruit juice or contain very juicy fruit bits that will soften the flakes.

Food Prep Terminology

This section is all about cutting, grinding, and blending techniques that provide varied textures to your raw snack recipes. Each task is simple to perform and requires only a brief explanation for comprehension and clarity. I provide this list here merely for those of you who are relative newcomers to the kitchen environment. Please note that these are my definitions that apply to the recipes found throughout this book. Other cooks and professional chefs may have slightly different meanings for these terms.

COARSELY OR ROUGHLY CHOP.
This is what you would do to fruits or vegetables if you were making a hearty, chunky, fresh fruit or vegetable salsa. The pieces are generally chopped no larger than ½ inch to ¾ inch square, with many of the pieces also being smaller, so that the recipe has plenty of varied textures. Coarse or rough chopping is done quickly, without precision.

CRUSH. The terms *smash* and *press* could alternately be used, but I generally use *crush* to refer to the processing of peeled garlic cloves when I want to reduce them to a mash before adding to a recipe.

CUT INTO CHUNKS. This is a general instruction for cutting food into whatever size easily fits into your blender, juicer, or food processor.

DICE. To dice an ingredient is to cut it into relatively precise cubes that should measure approximately ¼ inch to ⅜ inch square. Fruits and vegetables are often diced when making raw chutney, salad, marinade, or parfait recipes.

GRIND INTO A MEAL. I often use this instruction when the recipe calls for nuts, seeds, or oats to be ground into a medium or fine meal that is similar in texture to coarse or finely ground Parmesan cheese. You can use a nut and seed grinder to process small amounts, perhaps 1 cup or less, or a food processor to grind larger amounts.

Raw Foods Promote Life Force

The basic premise of "raw foodism" is that by nourishing your body with food that still contains its life force — that is, food that is replete with live enzymes, vitamins, minerals, amino acids, fiber, fatty acids, and sugars, in proper relationship and intact as intended by nature — you can potentially realize, in a relatively short period of time, a greater life force restored within your being. The benefits to your body include stronger immunity, increased general health, immense stores of energy, and greater longevity.

MINCE. To mince, or finely dice, means to chop or cut food into very, very small pieces of relatively uniform size — approximately $\frac{1}{16}$ to $\frac{1}{8}$ inch square. It is a process most often used with strongly flavored foods, such as garlic, onions, chives, ginger, and hot peppers, when you want to easily integrate a flavor into your recipe with minimal perceptible texture. A large chunk of ginger or jalapeño pepper used in a recipe can be a bit overwhelming if unexpectedly bitten into, but when minced and well incorporated, it adds a spicy essence. Use a medium to large knife. If you need a large quantity of food minced quickly, a food processor is the tool of choice.

LIQUEFY. I use the LIQUEFY button on my blender when I want to blend juices or nut milks with more-solid items such as soaked and softened dried fruits, nuts, seeds, or pieces of frozen fruit into a liquid, pourable consistency, thinner than a purée.

PURÉE. When making raw fruit or vegetable soups, frosty shakes, and some smoothies, most, if not all, of the ingredients are puréed, or blended in the food processor or blender until a thick or soupy consistency forms. The PURÉE button on the blender is often a medium speed. A puréed recipe is thicker in texture than one that has been liquefied.

SLICE. This is a very basic term that means to cut a relatively thin, flat piece or wedge from an ingredient such as a zucchini, carrot, bell pepper, potato, watermelon, or cucumber, or a loaf of bread or a pie.

SLIVER. To sliver a fruit or vegetable is to cut it into thin pieces approximately $\frac{1}{4}$ to $\frac{1}{2}$ inch thick or wide and 4 to 6 inches long, as you would when making bell pepper, carrot, cucumber, or summer squash strips or sticks. You don't have to be too precise with your measurements. Slivered foods are generally used as crudités and hand-dipped into pâtés, sauces, or dips.

ZEST. The zest is the thin, outer, colorful peel or skin of a citrus fruit that houses the flavorful essential oils. You can create zest by shaving or grating off the delicate, aromatic layer using a very sharp paring knife, zester, or file grater tool. Be sure not to penetrate down to the white, inner "pithy" layer beneath, as it tastes rather bitter.

Chapter 4

SUPER-SATISFYING

RAW NUT MILKS, SHAKES, SMOOTHIES, AND FROZEN FRUIT CREAMS

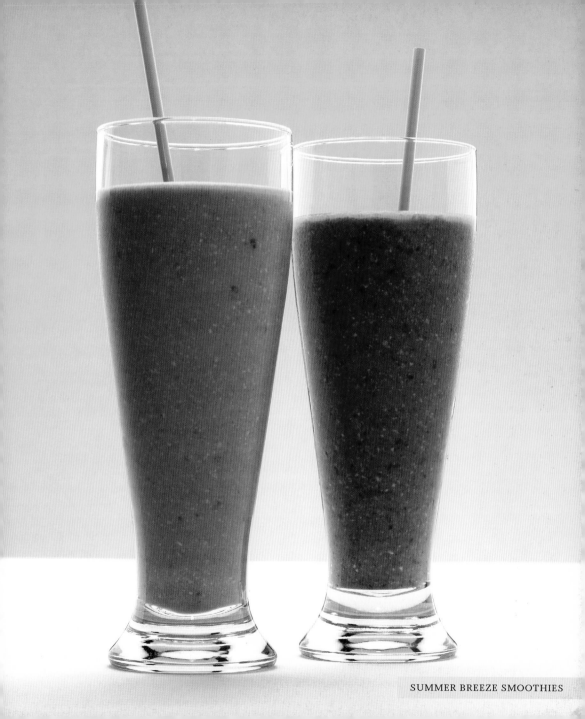

SUMMER BREEZE SMOOTHIES

This chapter deals with what I consider to be the most basic and essential of all raw snack food recipes — blender snacks. These favorite recipes make up the mainstay of my snacking repertoire. They are relatively quick and easy to make, and all you really need is a good-quality blender. Simply blend and pour, and out the door you go!

Unlike quickly digested, thirst-quenching, light-bodied, fruit and vegetable juices, which provide instant energy from their high natural sugar content, my shakes, smoothies, and frozen fruit creams are a bit heavier, containing virtually all of their fiber and a portion of carbohydrates, fat, and protein. They give you sustained, strength-building, fortifying energy for hours to come, and they satisfy on three levels: they're nutritionally dense and they satiate both appetite and taste buds.

The following recipes are perfect for growing kids or busy adults who need a lot of get-up-and-go power due to a physically demanding lifestyle. My blender snacks are delectable, easily digestible liquid mini-meals that maintain your energy for today's life on the run. If you don't have time to prepare a full traditional meal, substitute one of these recipes for a meal-on-the-go. You'll soon become a master at making these easy recipes, and you may even be inspired to create newfangled tastes and textures for yourself and your family.

NUT AND SEED MILKS

Homemade raw nut and seed milks are the vegan alternative to dairy milk. I highly recommend them as nutritious replacements for the pasteurized soy, almond, and rice milks that are now commonly available. Fresh, raw nut and seed milks, with their creamy flavor and silky texture, serve as an excellent base for smoothies, shakes, and frozen fruit creams and are delicious enjoyed alone or poured over muesli. These highly versatile drinks can be flavored and sweetened with foods such as dried figs, dates, prunes, raw honey, agave nectar, and even raw cacao or carob.

When making fresh nut milks, the more powerful your blender's motor, the better. Softened, soaked nuts must be thoroughly pulverized for the maximum flavor and nutrients to be extracted from the nut pulp.

Rich, silky, and slightly sweet, nut and seed milks contain a wonderful balance of protein, carbohydrates, and healthful fats, plus vitamins B and E and minerals such as magnesium, manganese, calcium, phosphorus, and potassium — nutrients that help to enhance memory and concentration, steady your nerves, and increase resilience to stress.

When stored in the refrigerator, the milk's yummy, rich "cream" will separate from the more watery portion and rise to the top. When this happens, simply shake vigorously for a few seconds to reblend prior to serving.

The pulp left over can be used for making dehydrated nut- or seed-based cookies or raw candy or fed to the birds and chipmunks as a special treat. It can also be composted if you don't want to eat it.

Raw Almond or Walnut Milk

If you're not already a fan of raw nut milks, I think you'll be pleasantly surprised by how fabulous they can taste, especially if you choose to use one of the sweetening options listed in the recipe below. If you or a family member is allergic to dairy milk, please give nut milks a try.

1½ cups raw almonds or walnut pieces

4 cups purified water

pinch of sea salt

sweetening options: 4 dried figs, stems removed; or 4 pitted medjool dates; or 1 tablespoon raw honey; or 1 tablespoon agave nectar. If using figs or dates, soak these in a separate small bowl overnight.

❶ Soak the nuts in a medium bowl covered by at least 1 inch of purified water for at least 8 hours. Drain and rinse.

❷ Place the nuts in a blender along with the water, sea salt, and a sweetening option, if desired. Blend on high for 2 full minutes.

❸ Strain the milk through a nut milk bag into a bowl. I do this in the kitchen sink. Using two hands, wring out the bag so that you extract every last drop of precious milk. This procedure may take a minute or so depending upon how thoroughly your blender pulverized the nuts.

❹ Transfer the nut milk to a quart-size liquid storage container. Store in the refrigerator for 2 to 3 days. It will also freeze quite nicely for future use. Shake vigorously before using, as the stored milk tends to separate.

Yield: 3 or 4 servings

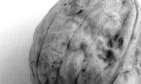

Cheater's Almond, Sesame, or Cashew Milk

Pressed for time but want a glass of fresh nut or seed milk? This recipe provides an easy way to "cheat" when making milk — no soaking and straining of nuts or seeds required. These milks are made with premade butters, available from your local health food store. They're lightly sweet, creamy, and rich in minerals, protein, and healthful fat. A small glass is energy-boosting and surprisingly filling.

2 cups purified water

3 tablespoons raw almond or cashew butter or sesame tahini

1 tablespoon raw honey or agave nectar

pinch of sea salt (optional)

¼–½ teaspoon vanilla extract (optional)

❶ Put the water, nut butter, honey, salt, and vanilla in a blender and blend on medium until smooth, about 30 seconds.

❷ Transfer the milk mixture into a liquid storage container and store in the refrigerator for 2 to 3 days. It will also freeze quite nicely for future use. Shake vigorously before using, as the stored milk tends to separate.

Yield: 2 servings

Cheater's Mexican Chocolate Almond Milk

Craving something rich, creamy, and chocolaty? This quick, delicious beverage will satisfy the kid in everyone. Raw cocoa, almond butter, and cinnamon blend together to form a smooth, indulgent yet highly nutritious beverage to add zip to your day. Great poured over a bowl of muesli, too!

For a spicy variation suitable for a holiday party, substitute a dash of nutmeg for the cinnamon and cocoa, and you've got a vegan version of raw holiday nog, sans eggs.

2 cups purified water

3 tablespoons raw almond butter

1 tablespoon raw cocoa (cacao) powder

1 tablespoon raw honey or agave nectar

dash of ground cinnamon

pinch of sea salt

¼–½ teaspoon vanilla extract

❶ Put the water, nut butter, cocoa powder, honey, cinnamon, salt, and vanilla in a blender and blend on medium until smooth, about 30 seconds.

❷ Transfer the nut milk into a liquid storage container and store in the refrigerator for 2 to 3 days. It will freeze quite nicely for future use. Shake vigorously before using, as the stored milk tends to separate.

Yield: 2 servings

SWEET AND LUSCIOUS: SMOOTHIES AND SHAKES

These recipes make my mouth water with anticipation! They're oh-so-yummy, ultra portable, and great for refilling your fuel tank when your energy gauge runs near empty.

My raw smoothies are lighter in calories and thinner in texture than shakes. These whipped, fruity, frothy, and refreshing drinks are perfect for when you're thirsty and slightly hungry, and your zippity-do-dah is beginning to get zapped but you don't want something too heavy. They're just what you need to keep the junk food temptations at bay.

My raw shakes are fabulously thick, frozen, creamy, and frosty. Unlike sugar-loaded dairy shakes, these indulgent snacks are nutrient-dense and filling. They contain a bit more fat, fiber, and heft than my smoothie recipes, and thus have more staying power to suppress your appetite and keep your energy flowing for hours on end.

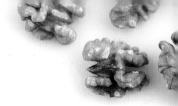

Creamy Banana Cocoa Shake

This sundae in a glass is full of health-building goodies that will make you feel invincible! It's super thick, so you may want to eat it with a spoon.

1 complete recipe of Cheater's Mexican Chocolate Almond Milk (page 100)

2 medium or 3 small frozen bananas, cut into chunks

⅓ cup raw walnut pieces

1 Put the milk, bananas, and walnuts in a blender and blend on medium until smooth and thick, about 20 seconds.

2 Pour into glasses or insulated mugs and enjoy.

Yield: 2 servings

A good source of: protein, omega-3 fatty acids, potassium, magnesium, manganese, phosphorus, B and E vitamins, fiber, and natural sugars

Brown Velvet Vigor Shake

This shake imparts concentrated fuel and bountiful flavors to stimulate your dynamic potential. I highly recommend it for those of you who expend a lot of physical energy during the day. It's quite replenishing. Consumed regularly, this shake is also a terrific natural treatment for chronic constipation. As a beauty bonus, the nutrients support glowing skin, hair, and nails.

2 cups purified water

8 pitted prunes (if hard, soak for 1 hour before blending)

2 medium or 3 small frozen bananas, cut into chunks

¼ cup raw oatmeal flakes

2 tablespoons raw tahini

1 tablespoon raw honey or agave nectar (optional)

pinch of sea salt (optional)

❶ Put the water, prunes, bananas, oats, tahini, and honey and salt if desired in a blender and blend on medium until smooth and thick, 60 to 90 seconds. Expect tiny bits of prunes and oat flakes in the finished shake.

❷ Pour into glasses or insulated mugs. This is a potent blend, so sip slowly. "Chew" each sip, mixing well with your saliva so that it digests with ease.

Yield: 2 servings

A good source of: age-defying antioxidants and B vitamins, plus potassium, phosphorus, magnesium, manganese, selenium, calcium, iron, zinc, protein, healthful fat, natural sugars, and fiber

Enzymatic Tropical Delights

If you want to receive yet another benefit out of your blended treat, you can add some pineapple or papaya to the mix. Both of these tropical fruits contain digestive enzymes — bromelain from pineapple and papain from papaya — that are critical to your health.

Digestive enzymes break food into particles small enough to pass through the intestinal wall and be absorbed by cells, where they are converted into energy. Beyond their role in helping your body break down, absorb, and assimilate the three basic components of food — carbohydrates, proteins, and fats — these enzymes have powerful anti-inflammatory, anticlotting, and antitumor properties. Because of these properties, I have found them to be an invaluable part of my medical practice, and I have used them in treatment programs for a variety of common health problems.

Digestive enzymes can also help reduce allergic reactions that some people have to certain foods. When a person lacks sufficient digestive enzymes, large molecules of incompletely digested protein can be absorbed through the small intestine. The immune system can't respond appropriately and reacts to improperly digested food as a foreign substance, which can trigger an allergic, inflammatory reaction. Digestive enzymes help reduce this inflammation.

— Susan Lark, M.D., in *Women's Wellness Today*

Orange-Apricot Blood-Builder Smoothie

Fresh, sweet, and tangy, this drink will fill you up and send your energy soaring. This is a wonderful blend to consume regularly if you suffer from iron-poor blood, as it offers the ideal mix of organic iron in the presence of vitamin C, plus copper: necessary nutrients for building red corpuscles in the blood, thus helping to relieve iron-deficiency disorders such as fatigue, anemia, pallid skin, and cold hands and feet.

10 dried apricots (if hard, soak for 1 hour before blending)

juice of 4 medium oranges, tangerines, or tangelos

¼ cup raw, hulled sunflower seeds

2 tablespoons raw tahini

❶ Put the apricots, orange juice, sunflower seeds, and tahini in a blender and blend on high until relatively smooth, about 60 seconds. Expect tiny bits of sunflower seeds and apricots in the finished smoothie.

❷ For a festive touch, set an orange slice onto the rim of each glass, pour in the smoothie, and insert an orange straw. This is a potent blend, so sip slowly. "Chew" each sip, mixing well with your saliva so that it digests with ease.

Yield: 2 servings

A good source of: antioxidants, vitamin C, and minerals such as copper, potassium, magnesium, manganese, phosphorus, calcium, iron, and zinc, along with a good dose of fiber, natural sugars, healthful fats, and protein

Green Gladiator "Go-Go" Shake

Although it contains algae, there's nothing fishy about this shake! Quite the contrary, this gently stimulating, blood-building shake is amazingly fruity and delicious. You'll see that I've added Siberian ginseng, also called *eleuthero*, which is one of the best herbs to use for increasing mental and physical stamina and endurance. This shake makes a wonderful breakfast, especially if you have a particularly mentally challenging morning ahead.

juice of 2 medium oranges, tangerines, or tangelos

2 cups frozen raspberries

¼ cup raw cashews or 1 tablespoon raw cashew butter

¼ cup purified water

1 tablespoon raw, unrefined coconut oil

1 tablespoon spirulina powder

2 teaspoons Siberian ginseng root (*eleuthero*) powder

❶ Put the orange juice, raspberries, cashews, water, oil, spirulina, and ginseng in a blender and blend on high until relatively smooth, 60 to 90 seconds. It will be very thick and fibrous. (If shake is too thick to blend with ease, add more water, up to ¼ cup.)

❷ Serve in glasses or insulated mugs. "Chew" each sip, mixing well with your saliva so that it digests with ease. Feel the power surge!

Yield: 2 servings

A good source of: potent antioxidants, vitamins B and C, plus potassium, phosphorus, selenium, magnesium, copper, iron, zinc, natural sugars, chlorophyll, easily assimilated protein, fiber, and healthful fats

Tangerine Dream Cream Smoothie

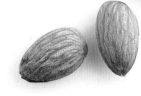

Simple and tangy, with a creamy citrus flavor, this shake is so lip-smacking good that it could be served as a nonalcoholic dessert drink!

1 cup almond or walnut milk (page 98)

juice of 2 medium oranges, tangerines, or tangelos

1 tablespoon raw, unrefined coconut oil

1 Put the nut milk, orange juice, and oil in a blender and blend on medium until smooth and frothy, about 30 seconds. Add a few ice cubes if you want it ultra frosty.

2 Pour into glasses and sip slowly, savoring the creamy tropical goodness.

Yield: 1 or 2 servings

A good source of: vitamin C, calcium, potassium, natural sugars, and healthful fat

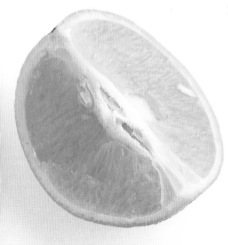

Summer Breeze Smoothie

Fragrant, fresh, and fruity, this smoothie hosts a medley of flavors that will tap dance on your tongue. This recipe makes an especially aromatic, gorgeous, light pink treat recommended for anyone who needs a constant flow of sustained energy.

1 cup purified water

1 cup fresh or frozen strawberries or raspberries

1 cup fresh or frozen peaches

¼ cup raw cashews or 1 tablespoon raw cashew butter

¼ cup raw oatmeal flakes

2 tablespoons raw honey or agave nectar

10 raw almonds

1 tablespoon raw, hulled sunflower seeds

1 tablespoon raw, unrefined coconut oil

❶ Put the water, berries, peaches, cashews, oats, honey, almonds, sunflower seeds, and oil in a blender and blend on high until relatively smooth, 60 to 90 seconds. Expect the texture to be fibrous with tiny bits of nuts, seeds, and oats.

❷ Serve in prechilled, frosty tumblers or wine glasses. Be sure to "chew" each sip, mixing well with your saliva so that it digests with ease.

Yield: 2 servings

A good source of: complexion-enhancing, stress-reducing antioxidants and vitamins B, C, and E, along with calcium, potassium, phosphorus, magnesium, manganese, copper, zinc, iron, selenium, fiber, protein, healthful fat, and complex carbohydrates

Peach Perfection Smoothie

Peach lovers rejoice! This dreamy, creamy smoothie tastes so scrumptiously grand, it will remind you of homemade peach ice cream. It is also an excellent nonalcoholic dessert drink.

2 cups almond or walnut milk (page 98)

2 cups super-ripe fresh peaches, peeled and cut into chunks, or frozen peach slices

1 tablespoon raw honey or agave nectar

2 teaspoons raw, unrefined coconut oil

pinch of sea salt

❶ Put the nut milk, peaches, honey, oil, and salt in a blender and blend on medium until smooth, about 30 seconds. Blend in a few ice cubes for an extra-frosty treat.

❷ This smoothie tastes so elegantly naughty and rich that it deserves to be served in your best glasses, sipped slowly and savored.

Yield: 2 servings

A good source of: antioxidants, vitamins B and E, calcium, magnesium, manganese, phosphorus, potassium, and healthful fats

Spicy Banana-Fo-Fana Date Shake

Satisfy your craving for sweets in a healthful way while building your body's inner fuel reserves. This shake will leave you feeling powerful and prepared for any possibility. Children love it!

1½–2 cups almond or walnut milk (use lesser amount for a frostier, thicker shake) (page 98)

4 Medjool dates, pitted (if hard, soak for 1 hour before blending)

2 medium or 3 small frozen bananas, cut into chunks

¼ teaspoon ground nutmeg or cinnamon

1. Put the nut milk, dates, bananas, and nutmeg in a blender and blend on medium until relatively smooth and thick, 30 to 60 seconds. Expect tiny bits of dates in the finished shake.

2. Pour into glasses or insulated mugs. Sip slowly and savor the luscious exotic flavor.

Yield: 2 servings

A good source of: natural sugars, potassium, sulfur, phosphorus, manganese, magnesium, iron, B and E vitamins, and fiber

Cantaloupe-Coconut Crush Slush

I like to refer to this slush, which is an icy cross between a shake and a smoothie, as my energizing beauty drink. It is relatively low in calories, and the bountiful beta-carotene — a nutrient that your body converts into vitamin A — helps to fight the effects of aging. Shredded coconut is optional but adds protein, texture, and more coconut flavor. It's incredibly thirst-quenching following exercise and perfect for when you want some light refueling.

1 medium cantaloupe, peeled, seeded, cut into chunks, and frozen

½ cup purified water or juice of 1 medium orange, tangerine, or tangelo

2 tablespoons unsweetened coconut, finely shredded (optional)

1 tablespoon raw, unrefined coconut oil

1 tablespoon raw honey or agave nectar

4 ice cubes

❶ Allow the cantaloupe to thaw for 20 to 30 minutes, depending on your kitchen's temperature, so that it is no longer rock hard from the freezer but still retains its icy texture.

❷ Put the cantaloupe, water, coconut, oil, honey, and ice in a blender and blend on high until smooth, about 30 seconds. Expect tiny bits of coconut in the finished slush.

❸ Pour into glasses or insulated mugs and relish the refreshment.

Yield: 2 generous servings

A good source of: fiber, potassium, folic acid, vitamin C, and beta-carotene

Morning Sunshine Divine Shake

This thick, creamy orange shake tastes like delectable ambrosia and has a lovely tropical aroma. It will enliven the senses and brighten a midwinter day, when citrus is at its sweetest, the weather is blah, and both your emotional and physical resilience have gone into hibernation. Active children, who need lots of sustained vigor — but who don't need refined sweeteners and subsequent hyperactivity — thrive on this shake.

½ cup raw cashews

juice of 3 medium oranges, tangerines, or tangelos

2 medium, super-ripe mangoes, peeled, pitted, and cut into chunks

1 tablespoon raw honey or agave nectar

❶ Soak cashews for 2 hours in enough purified water to cover by 1 inch. Drain.

❷ Put the softened cashews, orange juice, mangoes, and honey in a blender and blend on high until velvety and thick, about 90 seconds.

❸ Pour into chilled tumblers and delight in the silky smoothness.

Yield: 2 servings

A good source of: antioxidants, vitamins B and C, potassium, selenium, phosphorus, magnesium, copper, iron, zinc, natural sugars, enzymes, healthful fats, fiber, and protein

Blueberry Blast Shake

The flavonoids in blueberries help protect and strengthen the walls of the blood vessels and capillaries throughout the body and improve nocturnal vision. Blueberries aid in cleansing the blood and liver, help improve circulation, and have a mild laxative effect. I especially recommend wild Maine blueberries, preferred for their intense blueberry flavor, but any blueberries will be good. Young children, in particular, love this shake because it makes the tongue turn purple. If you want to avoid staining your teeth slightly blue, be sure to brush immediately after drinking.

1½ cups purified water

1 cup frozen blueberries

2 medium or 3 small frozen bananas, cut into chunks

2 tablespoons raw almond or cashew butter

1 tablespoon raw honey or agave nectar

1 Put the water, blueberries, bananas, nut butter, and honey in a blender and blend on medium until smooth, 30 to 45 seconds. Expect tiny bits of blueberry skin throughout this purple shake.

2 Serve in glasses or insulated mugs. Sip slowly, and feel invincible!

Yield: 2 servings

A good source of: youth-preserving antioxidants and energy-boosting nutrients such as iron, potassium, calcium, magnesium, manganese, copper, vitamins B, C, and E, protein, fiber, and natural sugars

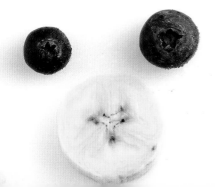

FROZEN FRUIT CREAMS

Totally vegan and totally fabulous, frozen fruit creams are decadent, full-fat, fruit "ice creams" with no dairy. These luxuriously creamy, super-thick desserts are specially designed for those of you who are very physically active, such as runners, high-mileage walkers, construction workers, landscapers, and aerobics instructors. To build and sustain all the energy you require, you need a healthy dose of calories packed with easily digestible proteins, natural sugars, beneficial fats, vitamins, and minerals, plus satisfying flavor.

The following recipes also make stupendous dessert treats for family and friends and serve as meal substitutes if desired. These are some of my favorite snacks to indulge in when I want something sweet, yummy, filling, heavenly, and good for my body, mind, and spirit.

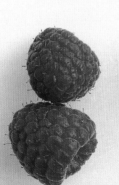

Banana-Chocolate Chip Frozen Fruit Cream

This sinfully delicious treat is an ultra-healthful banana-chocolate chip macaroon ice cream full of chewy bits of pure fuel that tastes of sweet indulgence. Think of it as ice cream with all of the good and none of the bad — it just doesn't get any better than this!

1 cup almond or walnut milk (page 98)

2 medium or 3 small frozen bananas, cut into chunks

⅓ cup raw cashews

¼ cup unsweetened coconut, finely shredded

2 tablespoons raw cacao nibs

1 tablespoon raw honey or maple syrup

1 tablespoon raw, unrefined coconut oil

1 teaspoon vanilla extract

pinch of sea salt

❶ Put the nut milk, bananas, cashews, coconut, cacao, honey, oil, vanilla, and salt in a blender and blend on medium for 30 seconds, then blend on high until the texture resembles thick ice cream, about 30 seconds longer. Expect tiny bits of coconut and cacao nibs throughout.

❷ Serve immediately in your favorite bowls, eat slowly, and savor the flavor. If the recipe is allowed to thaw a bit, it can be consumed as a shake.

Yield: 2 servings

A good source of: B and E vitamins, potassium, copper, phosphorus, selenium, magnesium, sulfur, manganese, iron, zinc, natural sugars, protein, healthful fat, and fiber

Cherry and Apricot Frozen Fruit Cream

Smooth, sweet-tart, and amazingly good for both your physical and psychological well-being, this velvety fruit cream is an invigorating snack.

- 1 cup almond milk (page 98)
- 5 dried apricots (if hard, soak for 1 hour before blending)
- 2 cups frozen cherries
- 1 medium or 2 small frozen bananas, cut into chunks
- 1 tablespoon raw honey or agave nectar
- 1 tablespoon raw, unrefined coconut oil
- 1 teaspoon vanilla extract
- pinch of sea salt

❶ Put the nut milk, apricots, cherries, bananas, honey, oil, vanilla, and salt in a blender and blend on medium for 30 seconds, then blend on high until texture resembles a deep burgundy-colored soft-serve ice cream, about 30 seconds longer. If your blender struggles with this thick mixture, turn it off and remove the lid. Using a long-handled spatula, stir to free the blades, add an additional splash of almond milk, replace the lid, and blend again. Repeat as necessary.

❷ Serve immediately in your favorite bowls, eat slowly, and savor the flavor. If the recipe is allowed to thaw a bit, it can be consumed as a shake.

Yield: 2 servings

A good source of: anti-inflammatory, antioxidant, and antiaging compounds plus iron, silicon, potassium, magnesium, manganese, vitamins B and E, protein, natural sugars, and fiber

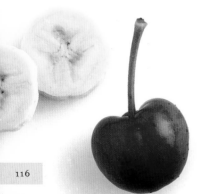

Strawberry-Citrus Frozen Fruit Cream

I rank this snack as one of my absolute favorites! It's light, luscious, smooth, and tangy-tart, resembling a fruit sorbet in color, taste, and texture. This peachy pink delight boosts your energy without weighing you down. Perfect for warm-weather snacking!

juice of 3 medium oranges, tangerines, or tangelos

2 cups frozen strawberries

1 medium or 2 small frozen bananas, cut into chunks

2 tablespoons raw almond butter

1 tablespoon raw honey or agave nectar

1 tablespoon raw, unrefined coconut oil

1 teaspoon vanilla extract

pinch of sea salt

❶ Put the orange juice, strawberries, bananas, almond butter, honey, oil, vanilla, and salt in a blender and blend on medium for 30 seconds, then blend on high until the texture resembles a soft sorbet, about 30 seconds longer. If your blender struggles with this thick mixture, add a splash of ice water to thin.

❷ Serve immediately in your favorite bowls, eat slowly, and savor the flavor. If the recipe is allowed to thaw a bit, it can be consumed as a shake.

Yield: 2 to 3 servings

A good source of: vitamins B, C, and E, potassium, calcium, magnesium, manganese, healthful fat, natural sugars, protein, and fiber

Chapter 5

FIT AND FABULOUS FRUIT AND VEGETABLE JUICES

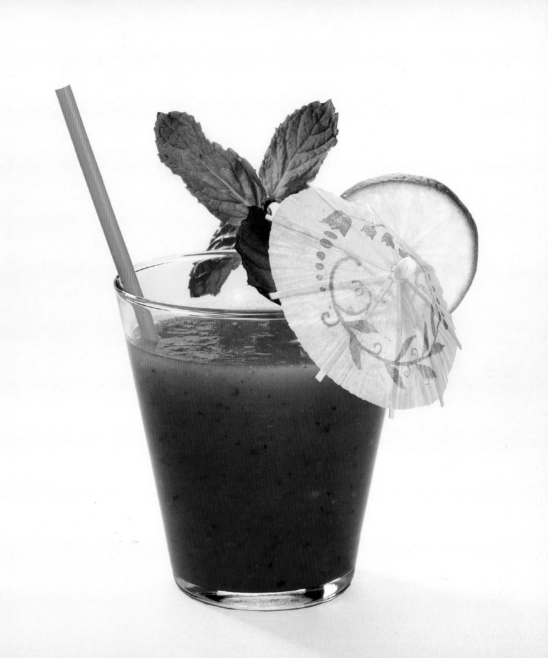

WATERMELON COOLER

Consuming real, fresh, raw juice has many benefits, aside from the pure gustatory delight of downing a colorful, fragrant glass of flavor. The action of a juicer breaks apart the normally indigestible cellulose pulp in fruits and vegetables, liberating more nutrients than would be available if those foods were simply chewed and swallowed. Drinking a daily glass of freshly extracted fruit or vegetable juice is a delicious way to obtain a portion of your necessary vitamins, minerals, enzymes, antioxidants, and daily fluid supply. As most of the fiber is removed during juicing, this luscious liquid, a concentrated source of natural sugars, is easily assimilated and provides nutrients on a cellular level within minutes. For the elderly or the infirm, or for one recovering from an illness, slowly sipping cool, fresh juices can be quite soothing and building to the system and can enhance vital nutrient uptake, especially if suffering from diminished digestive capacity.

Almost all juices available from the grocery store, whether in glass bottles, cans, plastic jugs, cardboard cartons, or aseptic boxes, are pasteurized (cooked) — read the label. Many contain added sugar, high-fructose corn syrup, artificial flavors, synthetic colors, undesirable artificial sweeteners, and preservatives and may be less than 30 percent real juice. Unless it says pure, fresh-squeezed or fresh-pressed, and unpasteurized, you can assume it isn't. Homemade juice or freshly extracted juice purchased from your local juice bar is the absolute best for your health and taste buds. Really fresh is what you want, not juice that's been sitting on the shelf for an unknown length of time.

If you are hypoglycemic or diabetic, I recommend that you dilute your juice by 50 percent with purified water. This will minimize the possibility of a "sugar rush" or "sugar high" that might throw your system off balance. This is the best way to serve juice to young children, as well.

JUICE BLENDS AND SINGULAR TASTE SENSATIONS

The following recipes are tasty juice blends derived from a variety of fruits and vegetables. But if satisfying, single-ingredient simplicity is what you are after, you can always whip up a fresh and frothy glass of pure carrot juice (one of my personal favorites), or try tart and tangy Granny Smith apple juice, or a potassium-packed glass of straight-from-the-garden tomato juice — a late summer delight here in my state of Maine. Remember, this book is all about integrating delicious, nutrient- and enzyme-rich, energizing snacks into your diet, so have fun, be creative, and don't be afraid to experiment with unfamiliar flavor combinations. You might be pleasantly surprised!

Note: Fresh juices oxidize quickly — in other words, their rich nutrient bounty rapidly diminishes with exposure to oxygen. Always drink fresh juices immediately after juicing to derive optimum benefit. As an alternative, though not the ideal way to consume fresh juice, minimal nutrient loss will take place if stored properly for a short period of time. So if you'd like to drink your juice several hours after making it for an energizing snack at work or school, or following a workout at the gym, simply store it in an airtight container such as an insulated beverage bottle immediately after making it, and keep chilled. Consume within eight hours.

V-5: Staying Alive Vegetable Juice Cocktail

Drink this daily for two weeks and I guarantee that your youthful vitality will spring forth once again. Your cells utilize the health benefits of this yummy "salad in a glass" almost immediately. If you consume an acid-producing diet (as most Americans do), heavy in meat, dairy, coffee, soda, and refined carbohydrates, then this is the drink for you. It will help to alkalize and normalize the body's chemistry.

4 stalks celery

½ medium bell pepper (any color), seeded, stem removed

6 medium carrots

2 medium tomatoes

1 medium cucumber

1 Juice the celery, pepper, carrots, tomatoes, and cucumber together.

2 Stir well before serving. Pour into glasses and enjoy.

Yield: 2 or 3 generous servings

A good source of: balanced vitamins and minerals, especially vitamin C, beta-carotene, folic acid, potassium, magnesium, calcium, silicon, and sodium

Here Comes the Sun

This vibrant juice beams with the colors of the sunrise and is simply chock-full of energetic vibrations that will strengthen and balance your innermost being.

3 medium oranges, tangerines, or tangelos, peeled and sectioned

3 medium carrots

1 ripe, medium papaya, seeded, flesh scooped out

1 Juice the oranges, carrots, and papaya, together. For this recipe, you don't need to use a separate citrus juicer for the citrus fruit — just toss it in with the other ingredients.

2 Stir to blend before consuming.

Yield: 2 servings

A good source of: vitamin C, folic acid, carotene pigments, potassium, calcium, natural sugars, and enzymes

Tart and Tangy Winter Nectar

Enjoy this midwinter blend when citrus fruits are at their best — succulent, ripe, and heavy with juice. Grapefruit is a great blood sugar stabilizer, and it helps to maintain energy and mood levels throughout the day. I especially like to serve this delightfully colorful beverage during the holidays.

- 2 medium pink or red grapefruits
- 1 medium lime
- 1 tablespoon raw honey
- 2 mint sprigs for garnish (optional)

❶ Cut the grapefruit and lime in half and juice with a manual or electric citrus juicer; strain out the seeds.

❷ Pour the juice into a blender, add the honey, and blend on medium for 10 seconds. Or vigorously stir room-temperature honey into the juice by hand.

❸ Serve in two of your best tumblers or wine glasses with or without crushed ice. Garnish with mint sprigs if desired.

Yield: 2 servings

A good source of: antioxidant flavonoids, vitamin C, and potassium

Body-Builder Cocktail

This juice blend is a bone-strengthening, muscle-building nutritional pharmacy in a glass. The generous chlorophyll content of parsley aids in the cellular uptake of oxygen, thus stimulating your metabolism. This is also the ultimate "beauty beverage" in that it promotes gorgeous skin, hair, and nails and relieves water retention throughout the body.

Note: *Due to parsley's natural kidney-cleansing properties, this strongly flavored blend can be a potent diuretic; don't consume more than 4 to 6 ounces per day.*

6 medium carrots

1 cup packed parsley (flat-leaf or curly), including stems

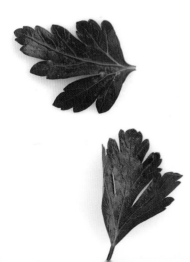

❶ Juice the carrots and parsley together. Use carrots to help push the parsley through the juicer if necessary.

❷ This is a very powerful juice. Please drink slowly, mixing each sip with saliva before swallowing. Don't chug it down or you might become slightly lightheaded.

Yield: *2 small servings, about 6 ounces each*

A good source of: calcium, iron, magnesium, sulfur, phosphorus, and potassium, plus bountiful beta-carotene, vitamins B and C, and energizing natural sugars

Watermelon Cooler (a.k.a. Virgin Pink Mojito)

Watermelon juice, naturally high in pick-me-up sugars, is the perfect choice to refresh, refuel, and rehydrate following a hard, sweaty workout or an afternoon spent mowing the lawn. This sensational, celebration-in-pink juice blend is also an excellent beverage to serve for alcohol-free summer entertaining. Sweet-tart and cooling to the palate, it looks especially enticing served in prechilled fancy glassware garnished with sprigs of fresh mint. For a festive option, add party appeal with colorful straws and tiny decorative umbrellas. Here's to summer!

4	cups cold, seedless watermelon, roughly cut into 1-inch chunks
	juice of 1 medium lime (about ¼ cup)
1	tablespoon raw honey or agave nectar
5-10	fresh mint leaves
2	mint sprigs for garnish (optional)

❶ Place the watermelon, lime juice, honey, and the 5–10 mint leaves in a blender. Liquefy until smooth and the mint leaves appear as tiny specks, about 30 seconds.

❷ Pour into two beautiful glasses with or without crushed ice. Garnish glasses with fresh mint sprigs, if desired.

Yield: 2 generous servings

A good source of: potassium, vitamin C, beta-carotene, and the cancer-fighting carotenoid lycopene

Morning Power Shot

This is my version of a spicy, ginger-flavored lemonade. Gingerroot is a pungent, moderately hot herb that enhances energy by increasing circulation throughout the body. Combined with a pinch of cayenne and vitamin C-rich lemon juice, this blend enlivens the senses, provides a rosy glow to the complexion, warms the body from head to toe, helps relieve indigestion, constipation, and motion sickness, and clears sinus and respiratory congestion. My Morning Power Shot will give you a bigger energy boost than you'd get from a shot of espresso — guaranteed! And with no caffeine jitters!

½ cup purified water

juice of 1 medium lemon (¼–⅓ cup)

2 teaspoons gingerroot, peeled, very finely minced

2 teaspoons raw honey

pinch of cayenne pepper

❶ Heat the water to just shy of a simmer in a small saucepan. Remove from heat.

❷ Put the lemon juice, gingerroot, honey, and cayenne in a medium mug and then pour in the hot water. Stir to blend and allow the mixture to steep for 4 to 5 minutes. The longer it steeps, the stronger and more potent the ginger becomes.

❸ Drink quickly, ginger bits and all, when the juice blend is comfortably warm. Feel the hot energy coursing through your veins! Raring to go now, aren't you?

Yield: 1 serving

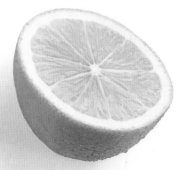

Apple Ginger Ale

This juice blend combines the core-warming, stimulating effects of flavorful gingerroot with the tart-sweetness of green apples. It gently increases circulation, tastes absolutely delicious, is full of potassium and pep-promoting natural sugars, and is a great, incredibly thirst-quenching pick-me-up for that afternoon slump. Nothing saps energy and strength more than indigestion and its accompanying painful and embarrassing symptoms: cramps, gas, headache, and bloating. Right? Consider this drink a cure for what ails you. Apple Ginger Ale makes a beautiful nonalcoholic light green treat for St. Patrick's Day or Christmas festivities. Children and adults will love it!

5 medium Granny Smith apples, including cores

1-2 thumb-size pieces of gingerroot (use the larger amount if you really like ginger's bite)

1 Juice the apples and gingerroot together.

2 Serve over ice and enjoy.

Yield: 2 generous servings

Vegetable Brain Blast

I enjoy this green blend on a regular basis for breakfast or as an afternoon snack. We don't generally think of our brain as requiring lots of energy, but it does. It consumes loads of fuel, especially carbohydrates, in order to perform at its peak. This beverage helps me maintain my mental stamina if I have a particularly trying task at hand that requires focused concentration. It also aids in the healing of acne, arthritis, and other inflammatory health problems.

3 medium apples, including cores

3 medium carrots

1 medium cucumber

4 teaspoons barley grass or wheatgrass powder

❶ Juice the apples, carrots, and cucumber together.

❷ Add 2 teaspoons of your chosen grass powder to each glass of juice and stir vigorously to blend.

Yield: 2 generous servings

A good source of: antioxidants, chlorophyll, potassium, calcium, silicon, trace minerals, and natural sugars

Old-Fashioned Apple Cider Vinegar Energy Brew

This drink was my grandfather's favorite afternoon pick-me-up. He was a farmer and routinely spent long, grueling hours in the hot Georgia sun tending to his crops and cattle. When he needed refueling and rehydrating but did not want anything too heavy weighing him down, he'd walk back to the house and quickly make this liquid refresher. It instantly replenishes the system, relieving fatigue, especially if you've been sweating profusely. He swore by its rejuvenating powers, due primarily to the natural sugars in the honey, enzymes and potassium in the vinegar, and hydrating property of water — a potent energizing trio!

Note: *Most commercially available apple cider vinegar is not raw. You need to look for the words* unpasteurized, unfiltered, *and* raw *somewhere on the label. Try Bragg Raw-Unfiltered Organic Apple Cider Vinegar, which is available at most health food stores.*

---

1 tablespoon raw apple cider vinegar

1 tablespoon raw honey

1 cup ice cold water

❶ Combine the vinegar and honey in a glass, stirring rapidly for 15 seconds or so until the honey is liquefied.

❷ Pour in the ice water and stir again. Drink quickly.

Yield: 1 serving

Post-Workout Replenisher

As you exercise and work up a healthy sweat, your body begins to deplete its stores of sodium, potassium, water, and glycogen (sugar), among other nutrients, and needs refueling when you've finished. Unlike sugary "energy drinks," this simple juice blend replenishes your body's spent vitality without being too sweet.

3 medium apples, including cores

3 medium carrots

2 stalks celery

1. Juice the apples, carrots, and celery, together.

2. Stir before serving. Pour into glasses and enjoy!

Yield: 2 servings

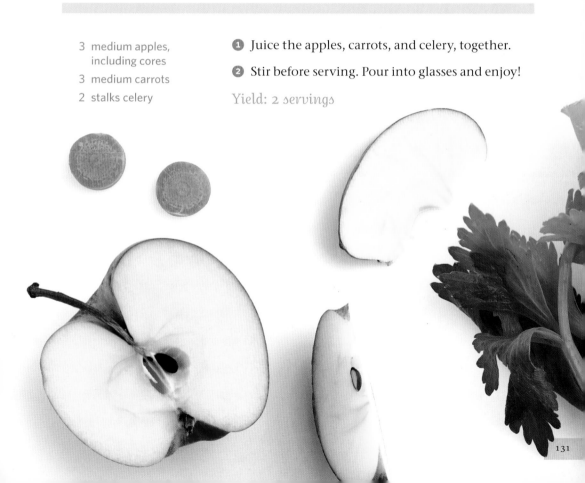

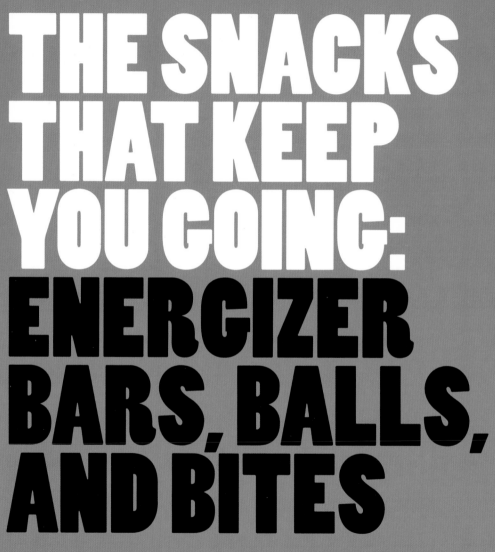

Chapter 6

THE SNACKS THAT KEEP YOU GOING: ENERGIZER BARS, BALLS, AND BITES

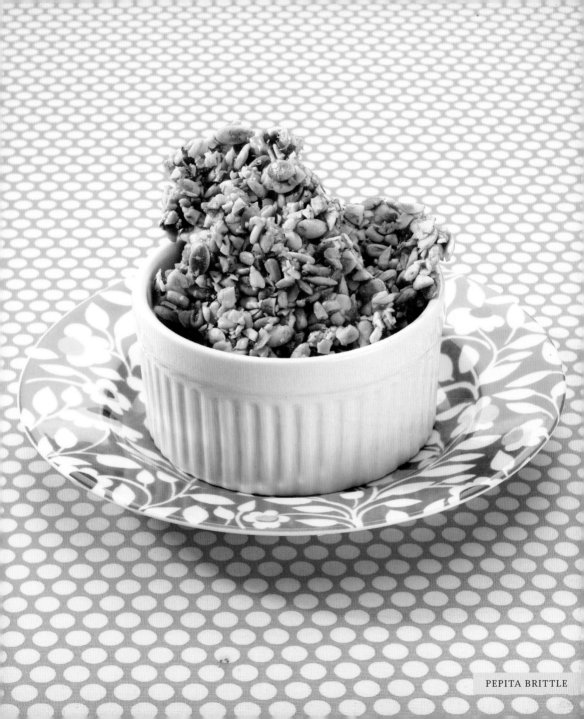

PEPITA BRITTLE

Ayurveda, India's ancient system of natural medicine, teaches of *ojas,* the essence of life that represents the "core" or "root" strength of the body and inherent immunity; the seed of nourishment and creativity; and the vital energy that is stored deep within the body. It is believed that *ojas* is the first thing to be created in the body of all living beings and that each is born with a certain allotment of *ojas,* be it a little, an average amount, or a lot, if you're lucky. The meaning of *ojas* is similar to that of the English word *constitution,* in that it is sometimes said that people are born with either a weak constitution (low energy, vitality, or health) or a strong constitution (high energy, vitality, or health) and that they will always have a tendency toward one end of the constitution spectrum or the other throughout their lives.

If you suffer from a weak constitution or low *ojas* or have depleted your naturally resilient constitution or high *ojas,* then the recipes in this chapter are for you. They provide nutritional fortification and help depleted bodies rebuild lost vitality and inner life force.

The snack recipes in this chapter make potent little nutrient powerhouses — what I like to refer to as mini energy meals for the potential athlete in all of us. Overflowing with grounding and building whole food ingredients — generally a combination of nut or seed butters, ground nuts, dried fruits, spices, and herbs — these tasty, sweet, filling, satisfying snacks will keep you going. Tuck one into your purse, briefcase, backpack, or gym bag so that you can snack when your energy flags or when you simply get a hankering for a delectable, rich, healthful morsel.

D L Many of the recipes in this chapter use a dehydrator. The icons above the recipe name indicate how much drying time you should allow for before your snack is ready.

Banana-Honey Granola Bars

Chewy and filling, a granola bar is perfect when you need a delicious lift or a snack to enhance athletic performance. These bars make a great breakfast, as they really stick to your ribs!

1 medium, very ripe banana, peeled

2 cups raw oat flakes

1 cup raw almond butter or natural roasted peanut butter

¼ cup raw honey

2 tablespoons bee pollen

1 teaspoon vanilla extract

1 teaspoon ground cinnamon

coconut oil, raw and unrefined

A good source of: complex carbohydrates, protein, healthful fat, fiber, vitamins B and E, and minerals such as potassium, phosphorus, calcium, iron, zinc, selenium, copper, manganese, and magnesium

❶ Put the banana, oats, nut butter, honey, pollen, vanilla, and cinnamon in a food processor or large bowl and blend or stir manually until you have a stiff, cohesive dough ball.

❷ Coat a 9-inch square pan with coconut oil and oil your hands as well. Pat the dough evenly into the bottom of the pan. Cover and place in the freezer for 24 hours so that the flavors can meld; the texture will become quite firm and chewy. Alternatively, you can roll the dough into bite-size balls if you wish, and store in the freezer as instructed below.

❸ Cut into nine 3-inch squares, then cut each square in half so that you have a total of 18 bars.

❹ Store the bars in a tightly sealed container in the freezer and consume within 2 weeks for the best flavor and texture.

Yield: 18 bars

Apricot Sunrise Salute Bars

These fruity bars offer a powerful combination of wholesome goodness — essential for boosting energy and robust health while building blood, bone, and immunity. Eaten regularly, they also help relieve chronic constipation and are highly recommended for growing children, teens, and women, in particular, who are often lacking in these vital nutrients.

1 cup dried apricots

¼ cup raisins

6 large dried figs

1 cup raw almonds

½ cup unsweetened coconut, finely shredded

pinch of sea salt

❶ Soak the apricots, raisins, and figs for 4 hours in enough purified water to cover by about 1 inch. Drain. Reserve the soak water and drink this refreshing, sweet fruit nectar later, if you wish. Trim any hard stem ends from figs and discard.

❷ Put the softened, soaked fruit in a blender and pulse on medium until you have a fruit paste. If your blender struggles, turn off the motor and use a spatula to free up the blades and repeat as necessary until desired texture is achieved. Scrape the fruit from the blender into a medium bowl. (Alternatively, you could use a food processor to make the fruit paste.)

❸ Grind the almonds into a medium-fine meal using a nut and seed grinder. Add the almond meal, coconut, and salt to the fruit paste and stir to blend

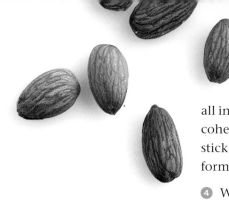

all ingredients. Mix thoroughly until you have a cohesive ball. The dough will be sticky, but it won't stick to your hands too much; you should be able to form bars with ease.

4 With your hands, form bars about 3½ inches long by 1½ inches wide by ¾ inch thick. Place them on mesh dehydrator screens, allowing at least 1 inch between pieces. Dehydrate at 105°F (41°C) for 18 to 22 hours. When the bars have reached the degree of density, moisture, and chewiness you desire, remove the screens from the dehydrator and allow the bars to cool for 20 to 30 minutes. They will become firmer as they cool.

5 Store the bars in a tightly sealed container in the refrigerator for up to 2 weeks or at room temperature for up to 1 week — if they last that long! These are perfect portable snacks to pack in your purse, gym bag, briefcase, or backpack, as they won't soften too much or melt in the heat.

Yield: About 12 bars

A good source of: antioxidants, vitamins B and E, calcium, magnesium, manganese, iron, boron, potassium, phosphorus, zinc, protein, natural sugars, healthful fat, and fiber

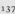

Get-Up-and-Go Apple-Walnut Bars

With the flavor and fragrance of apple pie and the chewy texture of cookies, you'll swear these are baked, but they're not. These are perfect snacks to pack in your purse, gym bag, briefcase, or back-pack, as they won't soften or melt in the heat. Eating just one is never enough — they're that good!

5-6 medium apples (firm varieties work best)

2 cups raw walnuts

1 cup raisins or currants

½ cup raw agave nectar

1 tablespoon ground cinnamon

½ teaspoon sea salt

❶ Core the apples. If they are waxed, you may wish to peel them; otherwise, leave the skins on for an extra dose of fiber. Grate, using a hand grater or food processor, until you have 3 full cups.

❷ Grind the walnuts to a medium-coarse meal in a food processor or nut and seed grinder. Sometimes I simply chop them in a nut chopper, as I like big chunks in this recipe, but it's up to you.

❸ Put the apples, walnuts, raisins, agave, cinnamon, and salt in a large bowl and stir well to blend. The mixture will be wet.

A good source of: antioxidants, potassium, calcium, copper, magnesium, phosphorus, iron, zinc, manganese, boron, protein, natural sugars, B vitamins, fiber, protein, and essential omega-3 fatty acids

4 With your hands, form bars about 2 inches wide by 3 inches long by 1 inch thick. As you form the bars, squeeze excess liquid back into the bowl; the bars should not be dripping when you set them on mesh dehydrator screens. Place the bars on the screens, allowing at least 1 inch between pieces. Dehydrate at 105°F (41°C) for 20 to 24 hours. When the bars have reached the degree of density, moisture, and chewiness you desire, remove the screens from the dehydrator and allow the bars to cool for 20 to 30 minutes. The bars will become firmer as they cool.

5 Store the bars in a tightly sealed container in the refrigerator for up to 2 weeks or at room temperature for up to 1 week.

Note: There will be some residual spicy "apple juice" left in the mixing bowl after forming all of the bars. It's really yummy and ultra-sweet, so don't waste it. Try it poured over muesli for breakfast the next morning.

Yield: About 12 bars

Pepita Brittle

This is my healthful, raw version of peanut brittle, without the tooth-chipping hardness, refined sugar, and corn syrup. It still delivers that satisfying combo of salty sweetness with lots of crunch. These snack bites pack quite a nutritional wallop that promotes skin, hair, nail, and prostate health and restores iron-deficient blood. Pepita Brittle is a great afternoon snack to munch, especially if your energy reserves are running on empty and it's still a few hours before dinner.

1 cup raw pumpkin seeds (pepitas)

1 cup raw, hulled sunflower seeds

½ cup raw honey

½ teaspoon sea salt

❶ Soak the pumpkin and sunflower seeds for 4 hours in enough purified water to cover by about 1 inch. Drain the seeds into a colander and leave them to drip-dry for about 30 minutes.

❷ Put the seeds in a food processor. Pulse-chop for only a few seconds, until the seeds are cracked and broken but not ground into a meal. A blender will also work, though not quite as efficiently.

❸ Transfer the seed mixture to a large bowl and stir in the honey. Sprinkle the salt evenly over the mixture and stir to blend thoroughly. The mixture will have a granular, moist consistency and will not form a cohesive dough.

④ Using a spatula, gently spread half of the mixture on a mesh dehydrator screen, forming a square about ¼ inch thick. Repeat the procedure with the remaining mixture onto another screen. Dehydrate at 105°F (41°C) for 22 to 26 hours or until the consistency is similar to thick, slightly flexible leather.

⑤ Peel the brittle off the mesh screens and let it cool on waxed paper or a cake rack for about 30 minutes. It will harden as it cools and will be even firmer and quite crunchy within a few hours of storage. Break into pieces of varying sizes.

⑥ Store in a ziplock freezer bag either in the refrigerator for 2 weeks or at room temperature for 1 week. Pepita Brittle packs well and makes a great travel or hiking snack.

Yield: Varies, depending upon sizes of broken pieces

A good source of: iron, zinc, selenium, copper, calcium, potassium, phosphorus, magnesium, manganese, essential fatty acids, natural sugars, vitamins B, D, and E, protein, and fiber

Chewy Cherry Charger Balls

Tangy, sweet, energizing goodness, these balls are chock-full of peppy spices, including a small bit of cayenne pepper. You'll barely taste the heat, but you'll feel the zip and the increase in circulation that it provides.

1 cup raw almonds

1 cup dried, pitted cherries, sweetened with apple juice or unsweetened

1 cup raw almond butter

3 tablespoons raw agave nectar or raw honey

½ teaspoon ground cinnamon

¼ teaspoon cayenne pepper

pinch of sea salt

A good source of:
antioxidants, vitamins B and E, calcium, magnesium, potassium, phosphorus, zinc, copper, silicon, manganese, iron, healthful fat, natural sugars, protein, and fiber

❶ Grind the almonds to a medium texture in a food processor or nut and seed grinder. The almonds should look similar to very coarsely ground Parmesan cheese.

❷ Put the almond meal, cherries, almond butter, agave, cinnamon, cayenne, and salt in a medium bowl. Using a large spoon or your hands, thoroughly mix the ingredients until a cohesive dough is formed.

❸ Pinch off pieces of the dough and form into balls about 1¼ inch in diameter and set aside.

❹ For the best flavor and consistency, allow the balls to set for 24 hours before eating. Store the balls in a tightly sealed container in the refrigerator and consume within 2 or 3 weeks. They may be individually wrapped, using waxed paper or plastic wrap, and taken with you to enjoy as portable energy bites.

Yield: About 24 balls

Green Glow Spirulina Balls

These small balls of glorious go-go power pack a mighty punch of energy. They also encourage luxurious growth of hair, glowing skin, and shiny nails, plus help relieve chronic constipation and menstrual cramping, if eaten daily. Don't worry — you won't even taste the spirulina.

- 1 cup raw sesame seeds
- ½ cup raw carob powder
- ½ cup raw agave nectar
- 3 tablespoons spirulina powder
- 2 tablespoons bee pollen
- ½ teaspoon ground cinnamon

A good source of:
beta-carotene, vitamins B and E, potassium, phosphorus, calcium, chlorophyll, magnesium, manganese, iron, zinc, copper, slow-release carbohydrates, protein, healthful fat, and fiber

1 Grind the sesame seeds to a fine meal in a nut and seed grinder.

2 Transfer the seed meal to a medium bowl and stir in the carob, agave, spirulina, pollen, and cinnamon. Blend thoroughly until you have a stiff, cohesive ball; your hands work best here.

3 Pinch off small pieces of dough and roll into balls the size of large marbles, about 1¼ inches in diameter.

4 For the best flavor and consistency, allow the balls to set for 24 hours before eating. Store the balls in a tightly sealed container in the refrigerator and consume within 2 weeks. They may be individually wrapped, using waxed paper or plastic wrap, and taken with you to enjoy as portable energy bites.

Yield: About 20 balls

Herbal Energy Balls

These toothsome snacks are full of vigor-building nutrients and antioxidants. The gently stimulating herbs and spices combine with sweet, creamy, tart flavors to provide sustained energy in one small package. Herbalists recommend taking Siberian ginseng on a regular basis to increase stamina and endurance and restore vitality deep within your core.

1 cup unsweetened coconut, finely shredded

1 cup raw almond butter

¾ cup unsweetened dried cranberries

½ cup raw honey

2 tablespoons Siberian ginseng root (*eleuthero*) powder

½ teaspoon ground cinnamon

pinch of sea salt

❶ Set aside ½ cup of the coconut in a shallow bowl for coating.

❷ Put the remaining ½ cup coconut, almond butter, cranberries, honey, ginseng, cinnamon, and salt in a medium bowl and stir well to blend. I normally use my hands instead of a spoon to really knead the ingredients into a cohesive ball.

❸ Pinch off pieces of the dough and form into balls about 1¼ inches in diameter. Roll each ball in the reserved coconut to coat.

❹ For the best flavor and consistency, allow the balls to set for 24 hours before eating. Store the balls in a tightly sealed container in the refrigerator and consume within 2 to 3 weeks. They may be individually wrapped, using waxed paper or plastic wrap, and taken with you to enjoy as portable energy bites.

Yield: About 20 balls

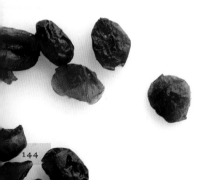

Bugs on a Log

Kids of all ages will love this simple little snack with the silly name. It offers a tasty twist with nutritional heft — transforming a serving of plain old unenticing celery sticks into a snack that melds salty, nutty, sweet flavors with chewy, creamy, and crunchy textures. They are quick to make and big enough to quell hunger pangs and rev up your engine.

2 celery stalks, ends trimmed

2-3 tablespoons natural roasted peanut butter or raw almond butter

¼ cup raisins, dried cranberries, currants, or fresh or dried blueberries

❶ Cut the celery stalks in half so that you have four pieces, each about 5 inches long.

❷ Fill the "valleys" of the celery stalks with your nut butter of choice. Press "bugs" (dried or fresh fruit pieces) into the nut butter. Enjoy!

Yield: 1 serving

A good source of: vitamin B, iron, zinc, potassium, calcium, copper, sodium, magnesium, manganese, phosphorus, antioxidants, protein, healthful fat, fiber, and natural sugars

Smooth Maple-Carob Zippers

Smooth as silk and delectable, these balls are a scrumptious, velvety, pop-in-your-mouth snack. They melt in your mouth and infuse your body with zing and zip, but enjoy these snacks at home: they are not easily portable, due to their soft consistency.

1 cup raisins

1 cup raw pecans

1 cup raw carob powder

3 tablespoons maple syrup

¼ teaspoon cayenne pepper

¼ teaspoon ground cinnamon

¼ teaspoon ground nutmeg

coconut oil, raw and unrefined

❶ Soak the raisins for 4 hours in enough purified water to cover by about 1 inch. Drain. The soaking water can be refrigerated and added to a smoothie recipe to serve as a sweetening ingredient later, if you wish.

❷ Put the pecans in a food processor and grind to a medium-fine meal. Add the raisins, carob, maple syrup, cayenne, cinnamon, and nutmeg and pulse-chop until you achieve a slightly chunky, fudgy consistency. Don't process to the point of a paste. The mixture will be very moist and thick, so you may have to use a spatula to free the blade a few times. Be careful.

❸ Scrape the dough into a medium bowl, then oil your hands with coconut oil.

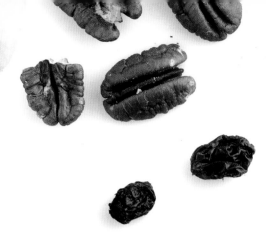

④ Pinch off small pieces of dough and roll into bite-size balls about 1 inch in diameter.

⑤ Store in a tightly sealed container in the freezer for up to 6 months. Wait 24 hours prior to consuming so that the flavors blend and the texture becomes firm and chewy. As these bites will be on the soft, sticky side if served at room temperature, I suggest eating them right out of the freezer while still chilled and relatively dry.

Yield: About 40 bites.

A good source of: B and E vitamins, antioxidants, calcium, potassium, phosphorus, iron, zinc, manganese, copper, magnesium, boron, fiber, protein, natural sugars, and healthful fat

Pecan Pick-Me-Up Bites

My husband simply adores these soft and chewy, bite-size morsels. Allergy sufferers should look for locally harvested bee pollen, as it can help relieve seasonal allergies. If you love the flavor combination of pecans and cranberries, these bites are a must-try!

2 cups raw pecans

1 cup dried cranberries, unsweetened

¼ cup raw honey

½ cup unsweetened coconut, finely shredded

2 tablespoons bee pollen

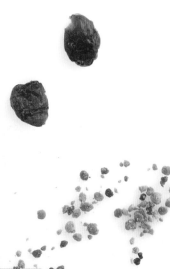

❶ Grind the pecans to a medium-fine meal in a food processor. Add the cranberries and blend until the entire mixture looks evenly granular and the cranberries are well incorporated, about 20 seconds.

❷ Pour in the honey, sprinkle in the coconut and pollen, and blend until the mixture forms a sticky, slightly oily, semigranular consistency that will easily stick together when squeezed in your hand. Scrape the dough into a medium bowl.

❸ Pinch off small pieces of dough and roll into balls about 1¼ inches in diameter and set aside. Gently press each ball between your palms to form small disks about 1½ inches in diameter.

❹ Place the disks on mesh dehydrator screens, allowing at least 1 inch between pieces. Dehydrate at 105°F (41°C) for 22 to 26 hours. When the bites have reached the degree of density, moisture, and chewiness you desire, remove the screens from the dehydrator and allow the bites to cool for 20 to 30 minutes. They will be soft when warm but will become much firmer as they cool.

❺ Store in a tightly sealed container in the refrigerator for up to 2 weeks or at room temperature for up to 1 week. These are perfect portable snacks to pack in your purse, gym bag, briefcase, or backpack, as they are so soft initially, but won't revert in the heat.

Yield: About 33 bites

A good source of: vitamins B and E, antioxidants, calcium, iron, copper, magnesium, potassium, phosphorus, zinc, manganese, healthful fat, natural sugars, protein, fiber, and antibacterial properties from the cranberries

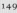

Chocolate-Orange Vibration Bites

Dark chocolate and fresh orange are a favorite combination, and both flavors are quite pronounced in these chewy, cookielike snack bites. Look to these yummies for gentle stimulation and increased circulation from caffeine and complementary spices, plus sustained energy from the raw oats. They're uncommonly good, so be forewarned; you could find yourself eating half the batch . . . like I did!

3 medium oranges, tangerines, or tangelos

1½ cups raw cashews

¼ teaspoon cayenne pepper

¼ teaspoon ground cinnamon

¼ teaspoon orange flavoring oil*

pinch of sea salt

1¼ cups raw oat flakes

½ cup raw cocoa (cacao) powder

¼ cup raw honey

coconut oil, raw and unrefined

❶ Zest the citrus fruit using a Microplane or the small holes of a box grater. You should have about 3 tablespoons of zest. Using a manual or electric citrus juicer, juice the oranges and set aside ½ cup of juice. Reserve the remaining juice for another use.

❷ Put the zest, juice, cashews, cayenne, cinnamon, orange oil, and sea salt in a blender and pulse on low to medium speed until you have a very chunky cashew butter. You may need to stop the blender a few times and use a long-handled spatula to scrape the bottom and free up the blades.

❸ Scrape the cashew mixture into a medium bowl. Add the oats, cocoa, and honey and use a spoon or your hands to thoroughly blend the mixture, forming a cohesive ball. The dough will be moist and sticky.

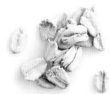

*Note: *Flavoring oil concentrations vary, so check your particular brand label for the correct amount to flavor 4 cups of food.*

④ Oil your hands with coconut oil so that the dough doesn't stick. Pinch off small pieces of dough and flatten into half dollar–size disks, about ½ inch thick. Place the bites on mesh dehydrator screens, allowing 1 inch between pieces. Wash and re-oil your hands as necessary while you work.

⑤ Dehydrate the bites at 105°F (41°C) for 13 to 15 hours. They will be dense and chewy when finished — similar to thick oatmeal cookies. Remove the screens from the dehydrator and allow to cool for 30 minutes.

⑥ Store in a tightly sealed container in the refrigerator for up to 2 weeks or at room temperature for 1 week. These are perfect portable snacks to pack in your purse, gym bag, briefcase, or backpack, as they won't soften or melt in the heat.

Yield: About 24 bites

A good source of: beneficial fat, vitamins B and C, antioxidants, protein, slow-release carbohydrates, fiber, potassium, phosphorus, calcium, sulfur, selenium, magnesium, iron, zinc, copper, and manganese

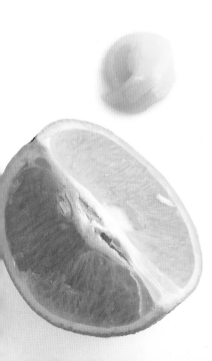

Power Balls

Unlike playing a lottery game such as Power Ball, where your odds of winning millions of dollars are slim to none, eating these Power Balls on a consistent basis will make you truly feel like a million bucks! These soft, sticky balls are too gooey to make good portable energy snacks; they are best eaten straight out of the refrigerator while still firm, chilled, and relatively dry.

1 cup raw almonds

½ cup crystallized gingerroot pieces

½ cup raw honey

2 tablespoons bee pollen

2 tablespoons Siberian ginseng root (*eleuthero*) powder

coconut oil, raw and unrefined

½ cup unsweetened coconut, finely shredded

❶ Grind the almonds to the consistency of a medium to fine meal in a food processor or nut and seed grinder.

❷ Dice the crystallized ginger into ¼-inch cubes.

❸ Transfer the almond meal and ginger to a medium bowl and add the honey, pollen, and ginseng. Use your hands to mash all the ingredients together until a cohesive ball is formed. The dough will be very sticky.

❹ Wash and dry your hands after mixing and then oil them well with coconut oil. Pinch off pieces of dough and roll them into marble-size balls about 1¼ inches in diameter. Set aside on waxed paper.

❺ Put the shredded coconut in a shallow bowl and roll each ball to coat.

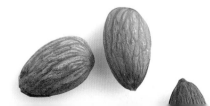

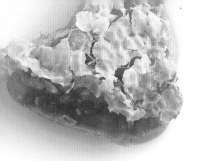

6 For the best flavor and consistency, allow the balls to set for 24 hours before eating. Store in a tightly sealed container in the refrigerator and consume within 2 or 3 weeks.

Yield: About 22 balls

A good source of: calcium, potassium, phosphorus, iron, zinc, manganese, magnesium, healthful fats, natural sugars, protein, vitamins B and E, and fiber, plus the pungent, warming bite of gingerroot and Siberian ginseng to increase circulation, and bee products — locally harvested if possible — which promote buzzing vigor

Figgy Waltons

Passionate about figs? These crunchy-chewy, super-sweet fig balls are my raw, healthful version of Fig Newtons. I highly recommend regular consumption of these tasty treats to encourage lustrous hair growth, strong nails, teeth, and bones, and also to help relieve constipation and symptoms of iron-deficiency anemia. The nutrients in these treats also promote balanced relaxation within the muscular and nervous systems; if eaten regularly, they help to relieve PMS cramping, sleeplessness, leg cramping, and restless legs. They are particularly energizing and rejuvenating pre- and post-workout. If you are concerned that you are not consuming enough calcium and other bone-building minerals, then you and these figgy delights should become best pals. They pack a wallop of fortification and protection.

1 cup dried figs

2½ cups raw English or black walnuts

1 cup unsweetened coconut, finely shredded

① Soak the figs for 4 to 6 hours in enough purified water to cover by about 1 inch. Drain the soak water into a glass, refrigerate, and enjoy this refreshing, sweet figgy nectar later if you wish. Trim any hard stem ends from the figs and discard.

② Process the walnuts to a medium-coarse meal in a blender, food processor, or nut and seed grinder. Expect the oily, moist nuts to stick to the sides and

A good source of: easily assimilated calcium, plus B vitamins, magnesium, manganese, phosphorus, iron, zinc, copper, omega-3 fatty acids, potassium, protein, natural sugars, and fiber

bottom of your appliance. Using a long-handled, flexible spatula, scrape the nut meal into a large bowl, then add the coconut.

3 Add the soaked figs to the blender or food processor you used to grind the nuts and pulse until you have a wet, chopped fig paste.

4 Add the figs to the walnut mixture; blend with a large spoon or your hands until a slightly sticky, cohesive dough ball forms. If it is too sticky, feel free to add more coconut, 1 tablespoon at a time, to stiffen the dough.

5 Pinch off small pieces of dough and roll them into marble-size balls about 1¼ inches in diameter.

6 For the best flavor and consistency, allow the balls to set for 24 hours before eating. Store the balls in a tightly sealed container in the refrigerator and consume within 2 weeks. They may be individually wrapped, using waxed paper or plastic wrap, and taken with you to enjoy as portable energy bites. Keep them cool and they won't soften too much.

Yield: About 35 balls

Lickety-Split Lifesaver Balls

This snack will refuel your energy tank while prolonging your life — sounds like a winner to me! If you like your snacks on the not-so-sweet side, then this recipe is for you.

1 cup unsweetened coconut, finely shredded

¾ cup dried, pitted cherries, sweetened with apple juice or unsweetened

½ cup raw almond butter

2 tablespoons raw honey

1 tablespoon raw cocoa (cacao) powder

1 tablespoon Siberian ginseng root (*eleuthero*) powder

1 teaspoon ground cinnamon

pinch of sea salt

❶ Combine the coconut, cherries, almond butter, honey, cocoa, ginseng, cinnamon, and salt in a medium bowl and stir to blend thoroughly, forming a chunky-textured, stiff, cohesive ball. Mix with your hands, if you like.

❷ Pinch off small pieces of dough and roll into balls about 1¼ inches in diameter.

❸ For the best flavor and consistency, allow the balls to set for 24 hours before eating. Store the balls in a tightly sealed container in the refrigerator and consume within 2 or 3 weeks. They may be individually wrapped, using waxed paper or plastic wrap, and taken with you to enjoy as portable energy bites — just be sure not to let them get too warm, or they will become very soft.

Yield: About 30 balls

A good source of: bone-, blood-, and body-building nutrients such as iron, potassium, calcium, magnesium, sulfur, phosphorus, zinc, copper, silicon, manganese, vitamins B and E, antioxidants, healthful fat, protein, natural sugars, fiber, and gentle stimulants derived from the addition of raw cocoa (cacao), cinnamon, and ginseng

Bites of Fruit and Nut Butter

Sometimes the most satisfying things in life are passed over because they are seen as too easy, too simple to be of value. Such is the case with this snack. It requires only two ingredients, a knife, and a couple of napkins, but its ease of preparation and abundance of flavor should make it a regular item on your snack menu. No-nonsense noshing!

1 ripe fruit of your choice: a banana, pear, or apple, or several strawberries

2-3 tablespoons nut or seed butter: almond butter, cashew butter, tahini, raw sunflower butter, or natural roasted peanut butter

Cut your fruit into bite-size slices. Smear each slice with a dab of nut or seed butter. Munch and enjoy! That's it — fortifying finger food at its finest!

Yield: 1 serving

A good source of: vitamins, minerals, protein, natural sugars, healthful fats, fiber, and energy-boosting power

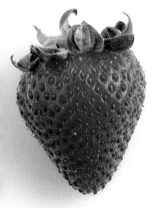

Shawn's Peanut Butter and Honey in a Cup

Growing up, my brother Shawn ate this twist on peanut butter and honey sandwiches nearly every day as his favorite after-school snack. Although I prefer raw almond butter, this is one of the recipes where I offer the option of a roasted peanut butter if your child or significant other resists raw nut butters.

You can make just a few tablespoons of this blend for quick, hunger-satisfying bites or mix up a half-cup batch — it's up to you. Eat it by the savory spoonful and let it melt in your mouth. This kid-friendly recipe makes an excellent snack paired with a glass of fresh almond or walnut milk (page 98) or fresh apple juice.

2 tablespoons raw almond butter or natural roasted peanut butter

2-3 teaspoons raw honey

Put the nut butter and honey in a small bowl or shallow cup and stir vigorously to blend until smooth and creamy. Eat up! What could be simpler?

Yield: 1 serving

A good source of: protein, filling fats, vitamins B and E, natural sugars, fiber, antioxidants, calcium, iron, zinc, copper, manganese, magnesium, potassium, and phosphorus

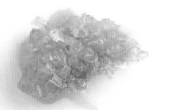

Almond-Raisin Cocoa Bites

Healthful chocolate? You bet! These are a dark chocolate-lover's dream! They're full of fabulous, sinfully delicious flavor — slightly bitter and not too sweet. These tasty little snacks energize, nourish, and provide a balanced form of energy; they're just right for popping into your mouth whenever you need a bite of power.

1 cup raw almond butter

1 cup dried currants or small raisins

½ cup raw cocoa (cacao) powder

3 tablespoons raw agave nectar or raw honey

1 tablespoon purified water

½ teaspoon ground cinnamon

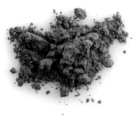

❶ Mix the almond butter, currants, cocoa, agave, water, and cinnamon with your hands in a medium bowl. Mash the mixture thoroughly, then form a stiff dough ball.

❷ Pinch off small pieces of dough and roll into bite-size balls about 1 inch in diameter.

❸ For the best flavor and consistency, allow the balls to set for 24 hours before eating. Store the balls in a tightly sealed container in the refrigerator and consume within 2 or 3 weeks. They may be individually wrapped, using waxed paper or plastic wrap, and taken with you to enjoy as portable energy bites.

Yield: About 42 bites

A good source of: heart-healthy fats, antioxidants, blood-building iron, boron, potassium, sulfur, calcium, zinc, copper, magnesium, phosphorus, manganese, vitamins B and E, protein, natural sugars, fiber, and gently stimulating caffeine, which increases circulation and blood flow

Manly Man Brazil-Nut Bars

These filling energy bars offer plenty of nutrients, they're not too sweet, and they have a pleasant mild flavor. I call them Manly Man Bars, but they're great for women, too! Regular consumption of these bars will encourage luxurious growth of hair and nails and promote clear skin.

2 cups raw Brazil nuts

½ cup dried apples

½ cup dried currants

¼ cup raw pumpkin seeds (pepitas)

1 cup unsweetened coconut, finely shredded

1 teaspoon ground cinnamon

pinch of sea salt

½ cup raw honey

❶ Soak the nuts, apples, currants, and seeds for 8 hours or overnight in enough purified water to cover by about 1 inch. Drain into a colander and leave the mixture to drip-dry for about 1 hour.

❷ Put the soaked ingredients, coconut, cinnamon, and salt in a food processor and blend until you have a nutty, granular consistency, about 30 seconds. Add the honey and blend again until you achieve a slightly sticky, moist, cohesive dough that will be easy to work with, about 60 seconds. Scrape the dough into a large bowl.

❸ Use your hands to form pieces of dough into bars that are about 3½ inches long by 1½ inches wide by ¾ inch thick and place them on mesh dehydrator screens, allowing 1 inch between bars.

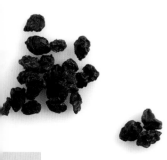

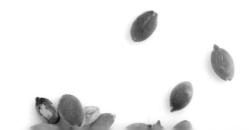

④ Dehydrate at 105°F (41°C) for 20 to 24 hours. When the bars have reached the desired degree of chewiness, remove the screens from the dehydrator and allow them to cool for 30 minutes. The bars will become firmer as they cool.

⑤ Store the bars in a tightly sealed container in the refrigerator for up to 2 weeks or at room temperature for up to 1 week. These are perfect portable snacks to pack in your purse, gym bag, briefcase, or backpack, as they won't soften or melt as long as they don't get too warm.

Yield: About 22 bars

A good source of: vitamins B and E, zinc, calcium, boron, selenium, copper, phosphorus, magnesium, iron, potassium, heart-healthy fat, natural sugars, protein, and fiber

Second-Wind Hazelnut Bites

Energy feeling low? Here's a pick-me-up snack that won't let you down. Hazelnuts and sunflower seeds add a rich crunchiness and smooth, mellow flavor to this yummy recipe. Especially recommended for prostate health maintenance, these hearty little snack bites will also support luxurious growth of hair and nails and prevention of PMS.

½ cup raw hazelnuts

¼ cup raw, hulled sunflower seeds

½ cup unsweetened coconut, finely shredded

¼ cup raw honey

¼ cup raw tahini

A good source of:
vitamins B, D, E, and K, selenium, calcium, potassium, phosphorus, magnesium, manganese, copper, zinc, iron, protein, essential fatty acids, natural sugars, and fiber

❶ Grind the hazelnuts and sunflower seeds into a medium-fine meal in a nut and seed grinder.

❷ Transfer the nut mixture to a medium bowl and stir in the coconut, honey, and tahini. Use your hands to blend the ingredients well and mash them into a small, cohesive dough ball.

❸ Pinch off small pieces of dough and roll them into bite-size balls about 1 inch in diameter.

❹ For the best flavor and consistency, allow the balls to set for 24 hours before eating. Store the balls in a tightly sealed container in the refrigerator and consume within 2 or 3 weeks. They may be individually wrapped, using waxed paper or plastic wrap, and taken with you to enjoy as portable energy bites.

Yield: About 23 bites

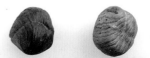

Frozen Banana Sundae Bites

These truly decadent treats taste like mini banana sundaes without the guilt of sugar and fatty ice cream! They will keep your energy soaring throughout the day and are great cooling snack bites to pop during the heat of summer.

½ cup raw hazelnuts

¼ cup raw carob powder

¼ cup raw agave nectar

¼ teaspoon ground cinnamon

3 medium bananas

A good source of:
loads of natural sugars, complemented by a nice supply of potassium, phosphorus, manganese, iron, fiber, calcium, zinc, copper, magnesium, B and E vitamins, and protein

❶ Grind the hazelnuts to a medium-fine meal in a nut and seed grinder and pour them into a bowl.

❷ Combine the carob, agave, and cinnamon in another medium bowl and stir thoroughly to blend. The consistency will be similar to chocolate syrup.

❸ Slice the bananas into ¾-inch-thick pieces. Roll each piece around in the carob mixture until coated, then coat again with a dip into the hazelnut meal.

❹ Lay the banana bites on a cookie sheet and place the sheet in the freezer, uncovered, to firm for 4 hours. Due to the high natural sugar content, the banana pieces will not become jaw-breakingly hard, but rather will be pleasantly firm and chewy.

❺ Store the bites in a tightly sealed container (ziplock freezer bags work well) in the freezer and consume within 2 weeks for the best flavor and texture.

Yield: About 24 bites

Chapter 7

POWERHOUSE NUT, SEED, AND FRUIT BLENDS

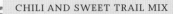

CHILI AND SWEET TRAIL MIX

Trail mixes have shed their reputation as hippie hiker food and become mainstream snack foods, enjoyed for their convenience, flavor, and nutritional benefits. Whether hiking, camping, biking, running, walking the dog, landscaping, gardening, tree-climbing, or pushing your child in a stroller, delicious trail mix is recommended for busy, on-the-go people who expend lots of energy in physically demanding jobs or exercise. It's also great for anyone who travels and wants to avoid fast food. These nutrient-dense, portable snacks pack easily in your purse, briefcase, auto, backpack, or gym bag and are loaded with sustained energizing goodness.

Nuts, seeds, and dried fruits are concentrated foods and calorically dense, so a little goes a long way and really satisfies. A quarter-cup is considered a single serving size. Remember to eat mindfully and slowly and to savor the flavors.

Why make these snacks yourself? When made in small batches at home, using only the best organic ingredients from a store with a high rate of ingredient turnover, you have total control of the flavor combinations and freshness. These aren't prepackaged snacks that have been sitting on a shelf for who knows how long.

The following assortment of simple-to-make recipes will satisfy a wide range of taste and texture cravings. There's a blend for everybody. Here's to your health . . . eat and be well!

D ◷ Don't forget to leave ample time for dehydrating when you see this icon!

Dynamite Trail Mix

This trail mix blend is pure nutritional dynamite, with just enough sweetness from the chewy apricots and zing from ginger's warming bite.

8 dried apricots

¼ cup crystallized gingerroot pieces

½ cup raw walnuts, whole or pieces

½ cup raw Brazil nuts

¼ cup raw pumpkin seeds (pepitas)

¼ cup raw, hulled sunflower seeds

pinch of sea salt

1 Cut each apricot into quarters. Dice the ginger into ¼-inch cubes.

2 Transfer the apricots and ginger to a medium bowl and mix in the walnuts, Brazil nuts, pumpkin seeds, sunflower seeds, and salt.

3 Store the trail mix in a tightly sealed ziplock freezer bag in the refrigerator for up to 6 months or in a dark, cool cabinet for up to 2 months.

Yield: 8 servings

A good source of: vitamins B, D, E, and K, antioxidants, omega-3 fatty acids, zinc, selenium, iron, manganese, magnesium, potassium, phosphorus, copper, calcium, protein, and fiber

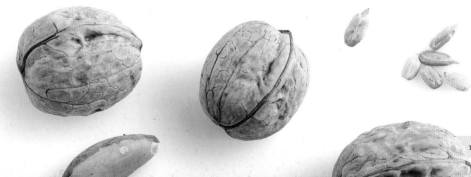

something to chew on

Banana Leather Bits

These chewy, dehydrated banana bits taste simply fabulous sprinkled on top of cold fruit soups, parfaits, or bowls of muesli and can be eaten with a spoonful of nut butter for a quick snack. It's tempting to consume the entire recipe at once, but keep in mind that one small handful equals one large banana.

6 large, ripe bananas, peeled

⅓ cup raw, unrefined coconut oil

A good source of: potassium, natural sugars, and fiber, along with a moderate amount of magnesium and B vitamins, plus healthful fat from the coconut oil

Note: This recipe fills my four-tray dehydrator. You may need to adjust the quantities of the ingredients for your particular dehydrator.

Yield: 12 servings

1. Slice the bananas into ¼-inch-thick rounds. Put the slices in a large bowl and pour in the oil. If the oil is solid or quite thick because your storage area is below 76°F (24°C), set the container into a pan of hot water until the oil liquefies.

2. Very gently toss and coat the banana slices with the oil. Be careful not to toss too much or the bananas will turn to mush.

3. Place the rounds onto mesh dehydrator screens and dehydrate at 115°F (46°C) for 22 to 26 hours.

4. Remove the screens from the dehydrator and allow the banana rounds to cool for 20 minutes. They will become more leathery as they cool. Bananas are loaded with moisture and will shrink considerably as they dehydrate, so don't be alarmed if the final quantity is a mere 6 handfuls!

5. Store in a ziplock freezer bag or other tightly sealed container for up to 2 weeks in either the refrigerator or a dark, cool cabinet.

D ⏱ 14–18 hrs

Cinnamon Maple Cashews

Crunchy, slightly sweet, with a little bit of chewiness . . . cashew lovers will adore this blend. Cashews are a bit lower in calories than other nuts and higher in energizing carbohydrates (sugars).

2 cups raw, whole cashews

1 tablespoon maple syrup

dash of ground cinnamon

pinch of sea salt

A good source of:
natural sugars, protein, heart-healthy fat, B vitamins, and several minerals such as potassium, phosphorus, magnesium, selenium, iron, zinc, and copper

❶ Soak cashews for 2 hours in enough purified water to cover by 1 inch. Drain the nuts into a colander and allow them to drip-dry for 30 minutes, then gently pat dry with paper towels.

❷ Transfer the cashews to a medium bowl and add the syrup, cinnamon, and salt; toss gently using a large spoon to coat. Try to avoid breaking the tender cashews.

❸ Using a slotted spoon, gently transfer the nuts onto one or two mesh dehydrator screens and dehydrate at 105°F (41°C) for 14 to 18 hours. Remove the screen(s) from the dehydrator and cool the nuts for 30 minutes. They will become crunchier as they cool.

❹ Store in a tightly sealed ziplock freezer bag in the refrigerator for up to 2 months or in a dark, cool cabinet for up to 2 weeks.

Yield: 8 servings

Sweet and Salty Trail Mix

Commercial nuts are often coated with an excessive amount of salt and sugar. Prior to dehydrating, the nuts in this mix are soaked in a diluted raw soy sauce and honey bath, allowing them to absorb just a bit of salty sweetness. This is one of my favorite blends. It keeps me going and really satisfies my salt-sweet tooth — healthfully!

- 3 tablespoons raw honey
- 3 tablespoons Bragg Liquid Aminos (raw soy sauce)
- 1 cup raw almonds
- ½ cup raw hazelnuts
- ½ cup raw pecans
- pinch of sea salt
- ½ cup dried currants

A good source of: calcium, iron, magnesium, manganese, antioxidants, potassium, phosphorus, boron, copper, zinc, vitamins B and E, heart-healthy fat, protein, fiber, and just the right amount of natural sugar from the chewy currants

❶ Stir the honey and soy sauce into 1 cup of purified water. Soak the almonds, hazelnuts, and pecans in the soy-honey water for 8 hours or overnight.

❷ Drain the nuts into a colander and leave them to drip-dry for about 30 minutes. Add a pinch of sea salt and toss the nuts to coat.

❸ Spoon the nut mixture onto mesh dehydrator screens and dehydrate at 105°F (41°C) for 18 to 24 hours. Remove the screens from the dehydrator and allow the nuts to cool for 30 minutes. They will become crunchier as they cool.

❹ Toss the nuts together with the currants and a dash more salt, if desired, and place in a tightly sealed container such as a ziplock freezer bag.

❺ Store in the refrigerator for up to 6 months or in a dark, cool cabinet for up to 2 months.

Yield: 10 servings

D ⏱ 22-28 hrs

Chili and Sweet Trail Mix

A mild mélange of zesty, slightly sweet flavors with amazing crunch, this pure nut trail mix is absolutely yummy! A handful of this mix, eaten when your energy stores are running low, provides true sustenance with staying power. It's also excellent when used as a salad topping instead of croutons.

- 1 cup raw pecans
- ½ cup raw almonds
- ½ cup raw Brazil nuts
- 2 tablespoons raw agave nectar or maple syrup
- 1 teaspoon chili powder
- ½ teaspoon cayenne pepper
- ¼ teaspoon sea salt

A good source of:
vitamins B and E, calcium, selenium, magnesium, potassium, phosphorus, manganese, copper, zinc, iron, protein, healthful fat, and fiber

❶ Soak the pecans, almonds, and Brazil nuts for 8 hours or overnight in enough purified water to cover by 1 inch. Drain the nuts into a colander and leave them to drip-dry for 30 minutes.

❷ Put the nuts, agave, chili powder, cayenne, and salt in a medium bowl and toss the nuts to coat.

❸ Using a slotted spoon, spoon the nuts onto one or two mesh dehydrator screens and dehydrate at 105°F (41°C) for 22 to 28 hours. Remove the screen(s) from the dehydrator and allow the nuts to cool for 30 minutes. They will become crunchier as they cool.

❹ Store in a tightly sealed ziplock freezer bag in the refrigerator for up to 6 months or in a dark, cool cabinet for up to 2 months.

Yield: 8 servings

Tropical Delight Trail Mix

Move over, Skittles and Starburst. This blend was designed especially as a healthful alternative to those addictive little candies for those of you with a chewy, tart-sweet tooth.

½ cup dried papaya spears or pieces, unsweetened

½ cup dried pineapple rings or pieces, unsweetened

½ cup dried mango slices or pieces, unsweetened

½ cup raw almonds

pinch of sea salt

❶ Tear or cut the papaya, pineapple, and mango into bite-size pieces and place them in a medium bowl.

❷ Add the almonds and salt and toss the ingredients with your hands or a spoon.

❸ Store in a tightly sealed ziplock freezer bag in the refrigerator for up to 6 months or in a dark, cool cabinet for up to 2 months.

Yield: 8 servings

A good source of: potassium, phosphorus, magnesium, manganese, zinc, iron, calcium, antioxidants, vitamins B, C, and E, healthful fat, protein, natural sugars, and fiber

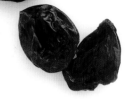

Summer Harvest Berry Trail Mix

Tart and chewy, slightly sweet, with a bit of crunch — I love the flavor and texture combination. This nutritionally fortifying blend is incredibly simple to make, and it's a great way to enjoy the flavor of summer berries throughout the year.

½ cup dried, pitted cherries, sweetened with apple juice or unsweetened

½ cup dried cranberries, sweetened with apple juice or unsweetened

½ cup dried strawberries, unsweetened

½ cup raw walnuts

pinch of sea salt

1 Combine the cherries, cranberries, strawberries, walnuts, and salt in a medium bowl and toss well to blend.

2 Store the mixture in a tightly sealed ziplock freezer bag in the refrigerator for up to 6 months or in a dark, cool cabinet for up to 2 months.

Yield: 8 servings

A good source of: antioxidants, vitamins B and C, potassium, iron, silicon, copper, zinc, magnesium, phosphorus, manganese, calcium, natural sugars, omega-3 fatty acids, protein, and fiber

Mighty Herculean Trail Mix

I can't guarantee you the brute force of a mighty Greek god, but with regular consumption of this blend, I can guarantee you more than enough energy to sail through your busy day. Bonus benefit: A handful eaten daily, followed by a large glass of water, will help relieve chronic constipation.

½ cup prunes

½ cup dried, pitted cherries, sweetened with apple juice or unsweetened

½ cup raisins

½ cup raw walnuts

dash of ground cinnamon

pinch of sea salt

❶ Cut the prunes and the cherries in half, if large, and remove pits if necessary.

❷ Combine the prunes, cherries, raisins, walnuts, cinnamon, and salt in a medium bowl and toss well to blend.

❸ Store in a tightly sealed ziplock freezer bag in the refrigerator for up to 6 months or in a dark, cool cabinet for up to 2 months.

Yield: 8 servings

A good source of: antioxidants galore, blood-building iron, zinc, copper, potassium, boron, silicon, phosphorus, manganese, magnesium, calcium, B vitamins, omega-3 fatty acids, protein, natural sugars, and fiber

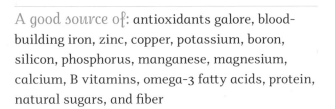

D ⏱ 10–14 hrs

Pepita and Sunflower Crunchies

It's nearing 3:00 p.m. and your energy gauge is running close to empty. If you're prepared and have this tasty snack at hand, you'll easily resist the nutritionally empty potato chips or crackers calling to you from the vending machine down the hall. These crunchies also make a terrific, tasty salad topping.

1 cup raw pumpkin seeds (pepitas)

1 cup raw sunflower seeds

1 tablespoon Bragg Liquid Aminos (raw soy sauce)

2 teaspoons extra-virgin olive oil

¼ teaspoon sea salt

A good source of:
vitamins B, D, E, and K, zinc, iron, selenium, calcium, copper, potassium, phosphorus, magnesium, manganese, healthful fat, fiber, and protein

❶ Soak the pumpkin and sunflower seeds for 4 hours in enough purified water to cover by 1 inch. Drain into a colander and leave the seeds to drip-dry for about 30 minutes.

❷ Put the seeds, soy sauce, oil, and salt in a medium bowl and stir well to coat the seeds.

❸ Spoon the seeds onto mesh dehydrator screens and spread evenly in a single layer. Don't allow the seeds to clump together or they will dry unevenly. Dehydrate at 105°F (41°C) for 10 to 14 hours. Remove the screens from the dehydrator and let the seeds cool for 30 minutes. They will become crunchier as they cool.

❹ Store in a tightly sealed ziplock freezer bag in the refrigerator for up to 6 months or in a dark, cool cabinet for up to 2 months.

Yield: 8 servings

Fig Lover's Trail Mix

Delectable figs, with their rich, sweet, alluring flavor, are great providers of energy, vitality, and nourishment. If you suffer from fatigue, PMS symptoms, constipation, or lackluster skin, hair, and nails, make this mix your friend. Your body and beauty will thank you!

1½ cups mixed dried figs (Black Mission, Turkish, and Calimyrna)
¼ cup unsweetened coconut flakes
¼ cup raw walnut pieces
pinch of sea salt

❶ Remove the stems from the figs and cut any large figs in half.

❷ Put the figs, coconut, walnuts, and salt in a medium bowl and toss well to blend.

❸ Store in a tightly sealed ziplock freezer bag in the refrigerator for up to 6 months or in a dark, cool cabinet for up to 2 months.

Yield: 8 servings

A good source of: calcium, potassium, iron, natural sugars, and fiber with lesser amounts of protein, B vitamins, copper, zinc, manganese, magnesium, and omega-3-fatty acids

Little-Known Figgy Fact

Intestinal parasites are destroyed by enzymes in raw figs, whether fresh or dried, but not cooked figs.

Hearty and Wholesome Trail Mix

This hearty and wholesome blend of raw ingredients is packed with interesting textures and flavors, and it's filling enough to stand in as a mini-meal. Need a quick breakfast? Put a quarter-cup of trail mix in a small bowl, toss in a handful of raw oat flakes, and top it off with fresh almond milk or pressed apple juice. It's a great way to start the day off right.

6 small dried Black Mission figs

½ cup raw almonds

¼ cup raw hazelnuts

¼ cup raw, hulled sunflower seeds

¼ cup raw pumpkin seeds (pepitas)

¼ cup coconut flakes, unsweetened

¼ cup dried cranberries, sweetened with apple juice or unsweetened

pinch of sea salt

1 Remove the stems from the figs and combine them in a medium bowl with the almonds, hazelnuts, sunflower seeds, pumpkin seeds, coconut, cranberries, and salt. Toss well to blend.

2 Store in a tightly sealed ziplock freezer bag in the refrigerator for up to 6 months or in a dark, cool cabinet for up to 2 months.

Yield: 8 servings

A good source of: antioxidants, vitamins B, D, and E, potassium, phosphorus, calcium, magnesium, manganese, iron, zinc, copper, selenium, protein, natural sugars, fiber, and healthful fats

Almond Crunch

The best way to enjoy almonds, in my opinion, is with minimal embellishment. Slightly sweet with a touch of cinnamon and salt, these crunchy nuts are wonderful served in a "nosh bowl" for company nibbles. They're so good, they'll disappear faster than a bowl of chocolate truffles — delectable almond simplicity!

½ cup raw agave nectar
1¼ teaspoons sea salt
2 cups raw almonds
¼ teaspoon ground cinnamon

A good source of:
calcium, magnesium, manganese, zinc, iron, potassium, phosphorus, vitamins B and E, protein, heart-healthy fat, and fiber

❶ Combine 1 cup of purified water with the agave and 1 teaspoon of the salt. Stir well to blend. Soak the almonds in this mixture for 8 hours or overnight.

❷ Drain the almonds into a colander and leave them to drip-dry for about 15 minutes. Sprinkle on the remaining ¼ teaspoon of salt and the cinnamon and toss the nuts to coat.

❸ Spoon the nuts onto one or two mesh dehydrator screens and dehydrate at 105°F (41°) for 28 to 35 hours. Remove the screen(s) from the dehydrator and allow the nuts to cool for 30 minutes. They will become crunchier as they cool.

❹ Put the nuts in a tightly sealed ziplock freezer bag and store in the refrigerator for up to 6 months or in a dark, cool cabinet for up to 2 months.

Yield: 8 servings

Mulberry Apple Walnut Trail Mix

If you've never tried dried mulberries, you're in for a treat; their flavor and texture remind me of fruity, chewy, milk chocolate candy. With regular consumption, your fingernails and hair will glow with health.

½ cup dried apples

¾ cup dried mulberries

½ cup raw walnuts, whole or pieces

¼ cup coconut flakes, unsweetened

pinch of sea salt

❶ Tear or chop the apples into bite-size pieces.

❷ Combine the apples, mulberries, walnuts, coconut, and salt in a bowl and toss well to blend.

❸ Store in a tightly sealed ziplock freezer bag in the refrigerator for up to 6 months or in a dark, cool cabinet for up to 2 months.

Yield: 8 servings

A good source of: potassium, phosphorus, magnesium, calcium, manganese, copper, iron, zinc, antioxidant flavonoids, boron, protein, omega-3 fatty acids, B vitamins, natural sugars, and fiber

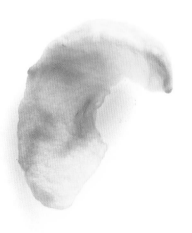

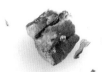

Chapter 8

RAW CEREALS AND DELECTABLE FRUIT PARFAITS

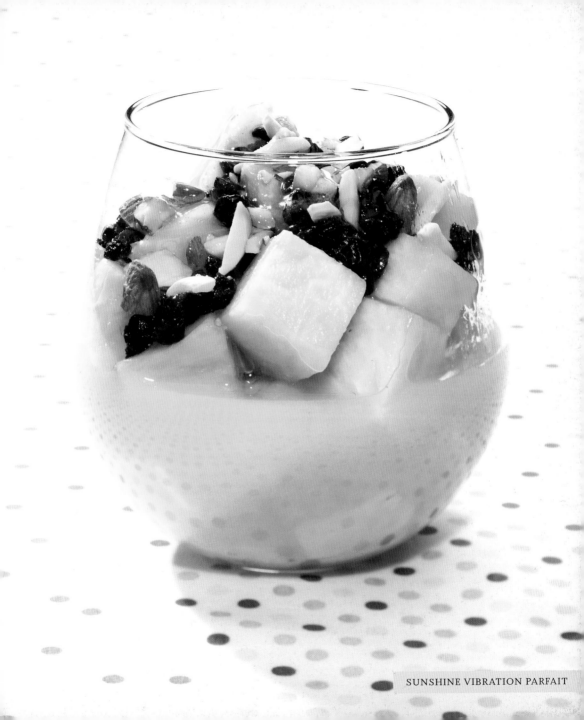

SUNSHINE VIBRATION PARFAIT

Cold cereal is a top pick for many folks who live life in the fast lane and must eat and run. Unfortunately, most supermarket brands are loaded with sugar, salt, and refined, puffed or rolled, processed grains. A good, hearty, whole-food-based raw cereal, often referred to as muesli, can provide a nutritious, soul-satisfying snack or even fill in for a complete meal if that's to your liking.

My raw cereals and fruity cereal parfaits are an interesting departure from what you'll find in a box. I like to blend raw oat flakes or soaked oat groats with dried and fresh fruits, an occasional drizzle of nut butter, coconut shreds, chopped or ground nuts, honey, and nut milks to make a variety of delectable delights. The following recipes are really quite delicious, even though they might sound a bit unusual upon initial review. I'm sure you'll find them super-tasty, filling, and fortifying.

Parfaits make the perfect breakfast for two. Eat slowly, chew thoroughly, and savor the flavors! If you'll be enjoying a parfait by yourself, go ahead and make the full recipe anyway. The second serving will keep, covered with plastic wrap, in the refrigerator for 24 hours.

Mighty Maine Blueberry Muesli

Living in the heart of Maine's wild blueberry country, I'm particularly partial to this muesli blend. It's easy to make and tremendously tasty eaten straight out of the container like a chewy trail mix or topped with fresh-pressed juice or nut milk and eaten as a raw cereal. This blend is quite filling and nutritionally dense; it's a perfect snack for someone in need of sustained energy.

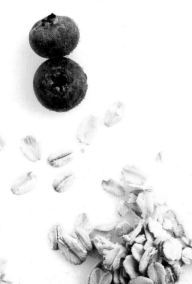

1 cup raw almonds

½ cup dried blueberries, sweetened with apple juice or unsweetened

½ cup raw oat flakes

pinch of sea salt

raw nut milk (page 97) or apple juice, to serve

❶ Put the almonds, blueberries, oats, and salt in a food processor and blend until the almonds are roughly chopped, about 20 seconds.

❷ To serve, top with fresh apple juice or your favorite raw nut milk and eat immediately, or cover the bowl and allow the muesli to soak, refrigerated, for several hours or overnight; the oat flakes will soften and the flavors will meld. Either way, it's delicious!

❸ Store the muesli in a tightly sealed container or ziplock freezer bag in the refrigerator for up to 6 months or in a cool, dark cabinet for up to 2 months.

Yield: 4 servings

A good source of: antioxidants, vitamins B and E, calcium, potassium, phosphorus, selenium, manganese, magnesium, iron, zinc, protein, slow-release carbohydrates, healthful fat, and fiber

Papaya and Pineapple Paradise Parfait

This recipe makes a spectacularly beautiful parfait to enjoy when the weather outside is damp and gray, your energy is flagging, and your mood is in the dumps. It's colorful and chewy and imparts fabulous fragrance and taste along with a dynamic nutrient load.

1 medium ripe papaya, seeded, flesh scooped out

1 cup raw pineapple, cut into bite-size pieces

½ cup raw almonds or pecans

¼ cup dried cranberries, sweetened with apple juice or unsweetened

¼ cup raw oat flakes

2 teaspoons raw honey

❶ Blend the papaya and pineapple in a food processor until puréed, 10 to 15 seconds.

❷ Process the nuts in a nut and seed grinder until very coarsely ground.

❸ Put the nuts, cranberries, oats, and honey in a medium bowl and stir to blend thoroughly.

❹ Layer the ingredients as follows into two wine glasses: put ¼ cup of the nut mixture in the bottom, then add one-quarter of the pineapple and papaya purée; repeat the layers.

❺ Enjoy immediately. If you're snacking solo, cover the second glass with plastic wrap, store in the refrigerator overnight, and eat it the next morning. It will keep for up to 24 hours.

Yield: 2 servings

A good source of: potent digestive enzymes and antioxidants, plus vitamins B, C, and E, manganese, magnesium, potassium, phosphorus, selenium, calcium, iron, zinc, protein, slow-release carbohydrates, healthful fat, and fiber

Apricot Marmalade

This versatile, spicy, sweet-tart, tangy spread can be used in all manner of ways with your raw snacks. For instant energy, eat it by the spoonful or mix a couple of spoonfuls with nut butter and a quarter-cup of your favorite trail mix for crunch. It works nicely as a sweetener in smoothies and shakes, as a fruit layer in parfait recipes, and as a topping on muesli.

2 oranges, tangerines, or tangelos

1 cup dried apricots

dash of ground cinnamon

pinch of sea salt

¼ cup dried cranberries, sweetened with apple juice or unsweetened

A good source of: potassium, iron, fiber, vitamin C, and antioxidants

1. Zest one of the citrus fruits with a Microplane or box grater and set aside the zest. Juice enough citrus fruit using a manual or electric citrus juicer to measure ⅔ cup.

2. Put the zest, juice, apricots, cinnamon, and salt in a small bowl. The apricots should be nearly covered by juice. Add enough purified water to cover the apricot mixture by about ½ inch. Stir well to blend.

3. Cover the bowl, refrigerate, and leave the apricots to steep for 8 hours or overnight.

4. After steeping, pour the apricots and any remaining liquid into a blender or food processor. Briefly pulse-chop until you have a chunky-smooth paste with the texture of marmalade. Scrape the mixture into a small bowl and stir in the cranberries.

5. Store in a tightly sealed container in the refrigerator for up to 2 weeks.

Yield: 1¾ to 2 cups

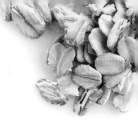

Autumn Glow Persimmon Pudding Parfait

The flesh of a very ripe, soft persimmon is a glorious, tropical sunset in reddish orange. Nothing compares to the tangy, sweet-tart flavor and smooth texture of this unique fruit.

2 large, very ripe persimmons

½ cup raw pecans

½ cup raw oat flakes

pinch of sea salt

almond milk (page 98), to serve (optional)

A good source of: antioxidants, vitamins B, C, and E, iron, potassium, phosphorus, calcium, selenium, zinc, manganese, copper, magnesium, protein, slow-release carbohydrates, healthful fat, and fiber

❶ Remove the tough stem caps from the persimmons and slice the fruits in half vertically, discarding the seeds. Scoop out the flesh as close to the peel as possible and put it in a food processor. Process for 10 to 15 seconds, until puréed. Alternatively, you could use a mortar and pestle and manually mash the flesh into a pulp.

❷ Process the pecans in a nut and seed grinder until very coarsely ground.

❸ Put the nuts, oats, and salt in a small bowl and stir to blend thoroughly.

❹ Layer the ingredients as follows into two medium wine glasses: put one-quarter of the persimmon purée into the bottom of each glass, then add ¼ cup of the nut mixture. Repeat the layers.

❺ Enjoy immediately as is or top with a bit of fresh almond milk. If you're snacking solo, cover the second glass with plastic wrap, store it in the refrigerator overnight, and eat it the next morning. It will keep for up to 24 hours.

Yield: 2 servings

Cranberry-Pecan Muesli

This muesli, my fall seasonal favorite, blends a winning combination of crunchy and chewy textures with tart and smooth. This delectable raw cereal will put a spring in your step and enhance your mental potential.

1 cup raw pecans

½ cup dried cranberries, sweetened with apple juice or unsweetened

½ cup raw oat flakes

pinch of sea salt

raw nut milk (page 97) or apple juice, to serve

1. Put the pecans, cranberries, oats, and salt in a food processor and process until the pecans are roughly chopped, about 20 seconds.

2. To serve, top with your favorite raw nut milk or fresh apple juice and eat immediately, or cover the bowl and allow the muesli to soak, refrigerated, for several hours or overnight; the oat flakes will soften and the flavors will meld. Either way, it's delicious!

3. Store the muesli in a tightly sealed container or ziplock freezer bag in the refrigerator for up to 6 months or in a cool, dark cabinet for up to 2 months.

Yield: 4 servings

A good source of: energizing nutrients such as potent antioxidants, vitamins B and E, potassium, phosphorus, selenium, manganese, magnesium, copper, iron, zinc, protein, slow-release carbohydrates, healthful fat, and fiber

Winter Fruit Muesli

This chewy, fruity muesli offers a mélange of flavors and textures that's bound to please even the most discriminating of palates. It's whole-food goodness guaranteed to keep you going!

¼ cup dried apples

3 Medjool dates

¾ cup raw oat flakes

¼ cup dried currants or small raisins

¼ cup raw sunflower seeds

¼ cup raw walnut pieces

dash of ground cinnamon

pinch of sea salt

raw nut milk (page 98) or apple juice, to serve

banana slices for serving (optional)

❶ Tear or chop the apples into bite-size pieces. Pit and chop the dates.

❷ Toss the apples, dates, oats, currants, sunflower seeds, walnuts, cinnamon, and salt in a medium bowl to blend.

❸ To serve, top with your favorite raw nut milk or fresh apple juice, add banana slices if desired, and eat immediately, or cover the bowl (sans banana) and allow the muesli to soak, refrigerated, for several hours or overnight; the oat flakes will soften and the flavors will meld. Either way, it's delicious!

❹ Store the muesli in a tightly sealed container or ziplock freezer bag in the refrigerator for up to 6 months or in a cool, dark cabinet for up to 2 months.

Yield: 4 servings

A good source of: vitamins B, D, and E, iron, zinc, copper, boron, selenium, potassium, phosphorus, manganese, magnesium, antioxidants, calcium, natural sugars, protein, slow-release carbohydrates, healthful fat, and fiber

Sunshine Vibration Parfait

Colorful, fragrant, refreshing, and uplifting to both mind and body, this fruity parfait is the perfect restorative snack to be enjoyed during a physically demanding day. Omit the almond butter and this luscious parfait is elegant enough to serve dinner guests as a light summer dessert.

1 cup raw pineapple, cut into bite-size pieces

1 tablespoon dried currants or small raisins

juice of 1 orange, tangerine, or tangelo (about ⅓ cup)

2 tablespoons raw almond butter

1 tablespoon raw honey

❶ Put the pineapple in a wine glass. Top with currants, then pour on the citrus juice.

❷ Drizzle the almond butter and the honey over the mixture.

❸ Eat immediately or cover the glass with plastic wrap, refrigerate, and enjoy up to 8 hours later.

Yield: 1 serving

A good source of: digestive enzymes plus vitamins B, C, and E, calcium, iron, zinc, boron, potassium, magnesium, manganese, phosphorus, natural sugars, protein, healthful fat, and fiber

Sweet Cashew Butter Drizzle

This citrusy, creamy sauce is a lovely pale peach color and has a delicious, buttery-sweet flavor. It can be enjoyed as a fruit dip or drizzled atop muesli or parfait recipes. So delicious is this butter, you must be careful not to give in to temptation and eat half the bowl in one sitting! Cashews are high in fat and slow-release carbohydrates, so indulging in a tablespoon or two of this treat will lift your energy, give you a bit of a power surge, and stave off hunger pangs for a while.

1 cup raw cashews

juice of 3 medium oranges, tangerines, or tangelos (about ¾ cup)

pinch of sea salt

1. Soak the cashews for 2 to 4 hours in enough purified water to cover by 1 inch. Drain and rinse.

2. Put the cashews, juice, and salt in a blender and blend on medium for about 30 seconds; increase the speed and "liquefy" for 30 to 60 seconds longer, until the mixture is smooth and creamy.

3. Store the nut butter in a tightly sealed container in the refrigerator and consume within 1 week for the best flavor and freshness. If the mixture separates, simply stir vigorously.

Yield: About 1¾ cups

A good source of: vitamins B and C, magnesium, calcium, phosphorus, potassium, iron, zinc, copper, selenium, healthful fat, natural sugars, and protein

Raw Fruit Compote

Making a bowl of dried fruit compote is a wonderful way to enjoy the ripe, sweet, succulent goodness of summer fruits in the dead of dreary winter. These particular dried fruits have an intense, hint-of-brown-sugar flavor. Feeling sluggish and irregular? Then this recipe is for you. It'll have you feeling zippy and back to your old comfortable self in no time.

½ cup dried Black Mission figs

½ cup dried apricots

½ cup dried cranberries, sweetened with apple juice or unsweetened

½ cup pitted prunes

pinch of sea salt

dash of ground cinnamon, nutmeg, ginger, or crushed cardamom pods (optional)

1 Remove the stems from the figs and put them in a medium bowl. Stir in the apricots, cranberries, prunes, salt, cinnamon, and enough purified water to cover by 2 inches. Soak the mixture on the kitchen counter until the fruits are nice and plump, about 24 hours. If the house is hot, cover the bowl and place it in the refrigerator.

2 Store the compote, including all the soaking juice, in a tightly sealed container in the refrigerator for up to 2 weeks.

Yield: 5 servings

A good source of: energizing nutrients such as iron, potassium, calcium, antioxidants, and natural sugars, plus a healthy serving of fiber

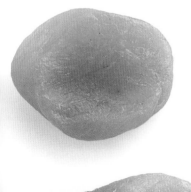

Living Strawberry Zipper Oatmeal

The ground strawberries lend a vibrant pink hue to this visually appealing cereal. Kids love it, not only because it's chewy and sweet-tart, but also because when it's topped with fresh almond milk, the milk turns pink. Don't let the cinnamon and cayenne combo scare you. The tiny amount of spice doesn't add heat, but it does increase circulation and blood flow throughout your body, adding a bit of zippiness to your step.

¾ cup oat groats

¼ cup raw almonds

1 cup fresh or frozen strawberries, unsweetened

½ cup raisins

2 teaspoons raw honey

⅛ teaspoon cayenne pepper

⅛ teaspoon ground cinnamon

pinch of sea salt

raw nut milk (page 97), to serve

❶ Soak the oats and almonds for 10 to 12 hours or overnight in enough purified water to cover by 1 inch. Drain and rinse.

❷ Put the oat mixture, strawberries, raisins, honey, cayenne, cinnamon, and salt in a food processor and blend until the oats and almonds are cracked and the mass has a moist, granular consistency, 20 to 30 seconds. Do not overprocess, or your cereal will turn into a paste.

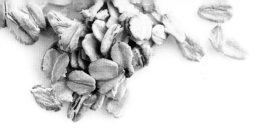

❸ To serve, top the cereal with your favorite raw nut milk and eat immediately, or cover the bowl and let the oatmeal soak, refrigerated, for several hours.

❹ Store the oatmeal in a tightly sealed container in the refrigerator for up to 2 days.

Yield: 5 servings

A good source of: antioxidants, vitamins B, E, and C, iron, zinc, potassium, selenium, calcium, boron, magnesium, manganese, phosphorus, slow-release energizing carbohydrates, healthful fat, protein, and fiber

Creamy Apricot Oaties

Smooth, sweet, and creamy, this heavenly blend of fresh and dried fruits, seeds, and oats is supercharged with wholesome power that will leave you feeling invigorated and ready to take on whatever life throws at you!

½ cup dried apricots
½ cup raw oat flakes
½ cup raisins
½ cup raw sunflower seeds
pinch of sea salt
raw nut milk (page 97), to serve
2 small bananas, to serve

❶ Cut the apricots into bite-size pieces and combine them in a medium bowl with the oats, raisins, sunflower seeds, and salt. Stir well to blend.

❷ To serve, top with your favorite nut milk and half of a small banana, thinly sliced. Stir to blend, mashing the banana pieces until a creamy consistency is achieved. Eat immediately or cover the bowl with plastic wrap, refrigerate, and eat a couple of hours later.

❸ Store the muesli in a tightly sealed container or ziplock freezer bag in the refrigerator for up to 6 months or in a cool, dark cabinet for up to 2 months.

Yield: 4 servings

A good source of: antioxidants, vitamins B, D, E, and K, iron, potassium, copper, selenium, boron, phosphorus, zinc, magnesium, manganese, calcium, healthful fat, protein, natural sugars, slow-release carbohydrates, and fiber

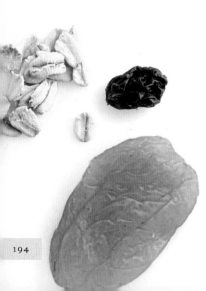

Mango Madness Parfait

This ambrosial parfait looks as great as it tastes and will promote a strong, vigorous, and resilient mind and body. Raw mangoes are a rich source of digestive enzymes. If you're snacking solo and don't have anyone to share the second parfait with, go ahead and pour on the almond milk, cover the glass with plastic wrap, store it in the refrigerator overnight, and eat it the next morning. I actually prefer the parfait when prepared this way, as the oats and coconut become quite soft and the flavors have a luscious, tropical goodness to them.

1 medium, very ripe mango

½ cup raw oat flakes

½ cup unsweetened coconut, finely shredded

dash of ground cinnamon

1 cup raw almond milk (page 98)

❶ Peel and pit the mango; cut the flesh into bite-size chunks.

❷ Layer the ingredients in two medium wine glasses as follows: 2 tablespoons oat flakes, 2 tablespoons coconut, then a layer of mango chunks. Repeat the layers. Top each glass with a sprinkle of cinnamon.

❸ To serve, pour ½ cup almond milk atop each glass. Soak for 20 to 30 minutes prior to eating to allow the oats to absorb the moisture.

Yield: 2 servings

A good source of: antioxidants, vitamins B, C, and E, calcium, phosphorus, selenium, manganese, potassium, magnesium, iron, zinc, protein, slow-release energizing carbohydrates, and fiber

Sweet Sustenance Muesli

If, like me, you're a fan of cherries and nuts, then you'll love this oat-free muesli — an extremely filling, luscious mélange of rich, sweet, and tart flavors accompanied by crunchy-chewy textures.

½ cup dried, pitted cherries, sweetened with apple juice or unsweetened

¼ cup raw almonds

¼ cup raw pecans

2 teaspoons maple syrup

pinch of sea salt

raw nut milk (page 97), to serve

1 small banana, for serving

1 Cut the cherries in half.

2 Grind the almonds and pecans with a nut and seed grinder until very coarsely chopped. Put the mixture in a small bowl.

3 Stir the cherries, syrup, and salt into the nut mixture.

4 To serve, top with your favorite nut milk and half of a small banana, thinly sliced. Stir to blend, mashing the banana pieces, until a creamy consistency is achieved. Eat immediately or cover with plastic wrap and eat a couple of hours later.

5 Store the muesli in a tightly sealed container or ziplock freezer bag in the refrigerator for up to 2 weeks.

Yield: 2 servings

A good source of: antioxidants, vitamins B and E, potassium, magnesium, manganese, copper, calcium, zinc, iron, silicon, phosphorus, healthful fat, protein, natural sugars, and fiber

Juicy Apple Muesli

This muesli is simple, filling, and reminiscent of an apple crumble, without the refined sugar and butter. This recipe makes a fabulously light, warm-weather breakfast or late-night snack. Kids love it!

1 medium, crisp apple

1 teaspoon fresh lemon juice

¼ cup raw oat flakes

1 tablespoon dried currants or small raisins

1 teaspoon raw honey

dash of ground cinnamon

pinch of sea salt

❶ Grate the apple, including the peel, into a medium bowl. Stir in the lemon juice to prevent the apple from turning brown.

❷ Add the oats, currants, honey, cinnamon, and salt to the apple mixture; stir to blend.

❸ Enjoy immediately, or cover the bowl and refrigerate for up to 8 hours or overnight, allowing the oats to soften and the flavors to mingle. It's delicious either way!

Yield: 1 serving

A good source of: vitality-building nutrients such as antioxidants, vitamins B and C, potassium, iron, zinc, phosphorus, selenium, manganese, magnesium, boron, natural sugars, protein, slow-release carbohydrates, and fiber

Cashew Currant Muesli

This is one of my all-time favorite muesli recipes. It's chewy, gently sweet, mildly flavored, and fabulous whether eaten right out of the bag or topped with freshly made apple juice. If your energy is flagging, it will definitely revive you until your next meal.

½ cup raw cashews

¾ cup raw oat flakes

½ cup dried currants

¼ cup dried blueberries, sweetened with apple juice or unsweetened

dash of ground cinnamon

pinch of sea salt

raw nut milk (page 97) or apple juice, to serve

❶ Process the cashews in a nut and seed grinder until coarsely ground. Transfer the nuts to a medium bowl.

❷ Add the oats, currants, blueberries, cinnamon, and salt to the cashews; stir well to blend.

❸ To serve, top with your favorite nut milk or fresh apple juice and eat immediately, or cover the bowl with plastic wrap, refrigerate, and let the ingredients soak and soften for a few hours or overnight.

❹ Store the muesli in a tightly sealed container or ziplock freezer bag in the refrigerator for up to 6 months or in a cool, dark cabinet for up to 2 months.

Yield: 4 servings

A good source of: vigor-building nutrients such as antioxidants, B vitamins, iron, zinc, boron, magnesium, manganese, calcium, phosphorus, potassium, copper, selenium, healthful fat, protein, slow-release carbohydrates, and fiber

Figgy Nut Muesli

Want to feel alive and function at your peak? Then this muesli is for you. It's tops for providing resilience and endurance balanced by a sense of calmness. Regular consumption of this muesli will improve the strength and sheen of your hair and nails plus help relieve constipation and strengthen bones.

1 cup dried Black Mission figs

½ cup raw almonds

½ cup raw oat flakes

pinch of sea salt

4 teaspoons raw honey

almond milk (page 98), to serve

A good source of: vitamins B and E, calcium, potassium, iron, zinc, phosphorus, selenium, magnesium, manganese, protein, natural sugars, healthful fat, and fiber

❶ Remove the stems from the figs and cut the figs into quarters.

❷ Coarsely chop the almonds in a nut and seed grinder; transfer to a medium bowl. Add the figs, oats, and salt to the almonds and stir well to blend.

❸ Drizzle 1 teaspoon of honey on each serving, then top with fresh almond milk. Enjoy the crunchy, chewy goodness immediately. If you want to soften the muesli, set the honey aside and cover the bowl with plastic wrap and refrigerate for a few hours. Add honey when you're ready to eat.

❹ Store the muesli in a tightly sealed container or ziplock freezer bag in the refrigerator for up to 6 months or in a cool, dark cabinet for up to 2 months.

Yield: 4 servings

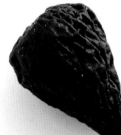

Creamy Banana Parfait

Sweet and chewy with a hint of tartness, this creamy parfait is one of my favorite snacks to enjoy after a strenuous power-yoga class. It healthfully satisfies a raging sweet tooth and that yearning for a snack that's smooth and creamy.

1 small ripe banana, thinly sliced

¼ cup raw oat flakes

¼ cup dried cranberries, sweetened with apple juice or unsweetened

dash of ground cinnamon or nutmeg

pinch of sea salt

almond or walnut milk (page 98), to serve

❶ Layer the ingredients into a medium wine glass as follows: put half of the banana slices into the bottom of a glass. Top with half the oat flakes, then half the cranberries. Add a quick dash of cinnamon and a smidgen of salt. Repeat the layers with the balance of the ingredients, omitting the spice and salt this time around.

❷ To serve, top with fresh nut milk and enjoy immediately.

Yield: 1 serving

A good source of: antioxidants, vitamins B and E, potassium, magnesium, manganese, selenium, phosphorus, iron, zinc, calcium, natural sugars, slow-release carbohydrates, protein, and fiber

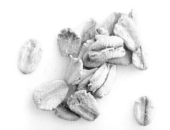

Living Raspberry Oatmeal

This is a beautiful cereal: the ground raspberries lend a vibrant, hot violet-pink hue to the entire recipe. Kids love the way nut milk turns pink when added to this cereal. In this oatmeal, the oat groats have been germinated (soaked), so they're alive and teeming with enzymes to help aid digestion.

1 cup oat groats

1 cup fresh or frozen red raspberries, unsweetened

½ cup raisins

2 teaspoons raw honey

⅛–¼ teaspoon ground cinnamon

pinch of sea salt

almond or walnut milk (page 98), to serve

❶ Soak the oats for 10 hours or overnight in enough purified water to cover by 1 inch. Rinse and drain.

❷ Put the oats, raspberries, raisins, honey, cinnamon, and salt in a food processor and blend until the oats are cracked and the mass has a moist, granular consistency, about 30 seconds. Do not overprocess or you will end up with an unappealing paste.

❸ To serve, top with your favorite nut milk and eat immediately, or cover the bowl and let the oatmeal soak, refrigerated, for several hours.

❹ Store the oatmeal in a tightly sealed container in the refrigerator for up to 2 days.

Yield: 5 servings

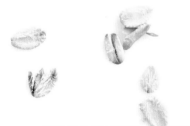

A good source of: antioxidants, vitamins B, C, and E, iron, zinc, potassium, selenium, boron, calcium, magnesium, manganese, phosphorus, slow-release energizing carbohydrates, protein, and fiber

Chapter 9

VEGETABLE JOLT: CRISPY CHIPS, ZIPPY DIPS, AND SCRUMPTIOUS SPREADS

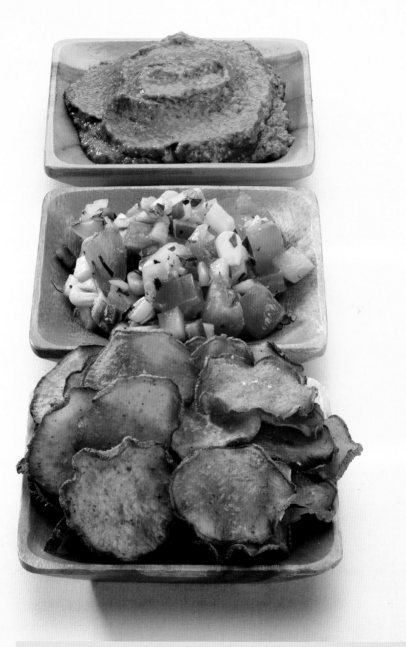

SWEET POTATO CHILI CHIPS, TEXAS TANGO SALSA, AND SPINACH-AVOCADO DIP

Raw vegetables are colorful, delicious, alkalizing, blood building, and mineral rich; will supercharge your energy stores; and can be eaten in a multitude of ways. There's no need to be limited to crudités or simple salads in order to fulfill your daily quota. Put an end to boring and bland and try my dehydrated chips, salsas, vegetable dips, and delectable spreads. The following recipes make great snacks, and entertainment foods as well. They're unique and so delicious that even your kids will be asking for more vegetables!

D ⏰ The vegetable chips all need plenty of time in the dehydrator. Be sure to look for the dehydration time icon and plan your time accordingly.

Ⓓ ⏱ 16- 20hrs

Zesty Zucchini Chips

These tasty chips provide another way to use this popular, prolific summer vegetable. I put my dehydrator through its paces when I have plenty of zucchini squash on hand. I think you'll be pleasantly surprised by the crunchy, concentrated, slightly sweet zucchini flavor that also packs a potassium punch plus beneficial antioxidants. These chips are the perfect "light munch" following a workout.

2-3 large zucchini (10–12 inches long)

1 teaspoon all-purpose or Italian seasoning herb mix

¼ teaspoon sea salt

¼ cup extra-virgin olive oil

Note: *This recipe fills my four-tray dehydrator. You may need to adjust the quantities of ingredients for your particular dehydrator.*

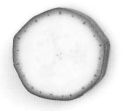

❶ Slice the zucchini into ⅛-inch- to ³⁄₁₆-inch-thick rounds. (The thicker the slices, the longer the dehydration process.)

❷ Place the zucchini rounds in a large mixing bowl and sprinkle with seasoning and salt; drizzle on the oil. Toss well to coat.

❸ Place the zucchini on mesh dehydrator screens so that the rounds are touching but not overlapping. Due to its high water content, zucchini squash will shrink considerably, so don't be alarmed if your finished chips look much smaller than you anticipated. Dehydrate for 16 to 20 hours at 110°F (43°C), or until crispy.

❹ Remove the screens from the dehydrator and allow the chips to cool completely for about 20 minutes. Store the chips in an airtight container in a cool cabinet for 1 week.

Yield: 3 or 4 servings

Sea Salty Yellow Squash Chips

These vegetable chips are similar to my Zesty Zucchini Chips, on the previous page, as far as nutrient content, crunch, and texture go, but I've seasoned them with only sea salt and pungent, freshly ground black pepper. They make a terrific salad topping, taste wonderful smeared with pesto, or, like the zucchini chips, are the perfect "light munch" following a workout.

4-5 large yellow summer squash (10-12 inches long)

½ teaspoon sea salt

½ teaspoon freshly ground black pepper

¼ cup extra-virgin olive oil

Note: *This recipe fills my four-tray dehydrator. You may need to adjust the quantities of ingredients for your particular dehydrator.*

❶ Slice the squash into ⅛-inch- to ³⁄₁₆-inch-thick rounds. (The thicker the slices, the longer the dehydration process.)

❷ Place the squash rounds into a large mixing bowl and sprinkle with salt and pepper, then drizzle on the olive oil. Toss well to coat.

❸ Place the squash on mesh dehydrator screens so that the rounds are touching but not overlapping. Due to its high water content, yellow squash will shrink considerably, so don't be alarmed if your finished chips look much smaller than you anticipated. Dehydrate for 16 to 20 hours at 110°F (43°C), or until crispy.

❹ Remove the screens from the dehydrator and allow the chips to cool completely for about 20 minutes. Store the chips in an airtight container in a cool cabinet for 1 week.

Yield: 3 or 4 servings

Spinach-Avocado Dip

This dip is alive with flavor and explodes with a wondrous emerald green vibrancy. It is tasty as a spread on sprouted Essene bread or flax crackers or used as a salad dressing. It can also be stuffed into a large romaine lettuce leaf, rolled up, and eaten as a vegan burrito.

1 ripe, medium Hass avocado

1 medium onion, roughly chopped (about 1 cup)

1 tablespoon fresh lemon juice

3 cups stemmed spinach leaves, tightly packed

1 teaspoon sea salt

❶ Slice the avocado in half lengthwise and remove the pit. Scoop the flesh into a food processor.

❷ Add the onion and lemon juice to the food processor along with the spinach leaves and salt. Process until relatively smooth, 60 to 90 seconds. Expect the texture to retain bits of spinach flecks and fiber.

❸ Store in a tightly sealed container in the refrigerator for up to 2 days.

Yield: About 2 cups

A good source of: blood-building iron and chlorophyll, plus antioxidants, vitamins B, C, and K, calcium, potassium, iron, magnesium, sulfur, slow-release carbohydrates, healthful fat, and fiber

Sweet Potato Chili Chips

These dehydrated — not fried — chips satisfy my craving for crunch, salt, and Tex-Mex flavor without grease or guilt. They promote clear skin, regularity, and good vision. Finicky eaters and potato chip-aholics will adore them and beg for more. Perfect to munch on the go and to take backpacking, as they are light as a feather yet keep your metabolism stoked.

2 large orange sweet potatoes

1 teaspoon chili powder

½ teaspoon sea salt

¼ cup extra-virgin olive oil

1 tablespoon Bragg Liquid Aminos (raw soy sauce)

1 Cut off the ends of the potatoes (no peeling required). Using a mandoline or spiral slicer, slice the potatoes into ¹⁄₁₆-inch-thick rounds. Try not to slice them much thicker than that or the chips will be too chewy, like sweet potato jerky.

2 Put the potato rounds in a large mixing bowl and sprinkle with the chili powder and salt, then drizzle on the olive oil and soy sauce. Toss well to coat.

3 Place the potato rounds on mesh dehydrator screens so that the rounds are touching but not overlapping. Due to their high water content, sweet potatoes will shrink considerably, so don't be alarmed if your finished chips look much smaller than you anticipated. Dehydrate for 15 to 18 hours at 110°F (43°C), until crispy or crispy-chewy. Their high sugar content makes sweet potato chips slightly chewier than white potato chips.

4 Remove the screens from the dehydrator and allow the chips to cool completely for about 20 minutes. Store the chips in an airtight container in a cool cabinet for 1 week or so.

Note: *This recipe fills my four-tray dehydrator. You may need to adjust the quantities of ingredients for your particular dehydrator.*

Yield: 3 to 4 servings

A good source of: antioxidants, vitamins C and B, potassium, iron, slow-release carbohydrates, and fiber

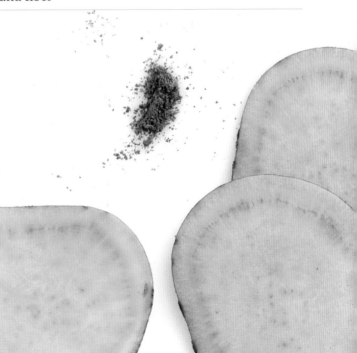

Texas Tango Salsa

Fresh, raw salsa is far superior in taste, texture, and vibrancy to its cooked, jarred cousin. There's just no comparison! Use this salsa to fill a large romaine lettuce leaf. Just roll it up like a burrito and you've got the ultimate vegan Tex-Mex snack! Also terrific eaten by the spoonful as a quick snack salad.

2 cups roughly chopped tomatoes

½ cup diced red onion

1 medium, yellow bell pepper, cored and diced (about 1 cup)

1 medium jalapeño pepper, seeded and minced

1 garlic clove, crushed

¼ cup cilantro leaves, tightly packed

½ cup raw corn kernels, fresh or frozen

1 tablespoon fresh lime juice

½ teaspoon ground cumin

½ teaspoon sea salt

½ teaspoon freshly ground black pepper

❶ Combine the tomatoes, onion, bell pepper, jalapeño, and garlic in a medium bowl.

❷ Finely chop the cilantro leaves. Add the cilantro and the corn to the tomato mixture.

❸ Combine the lime juice with the cumin, salt, and black pepper in a small bowl. Stir and then pour over the tomato mixture. Blend well with a large spoon.

❹ Store in a tightly sealed container in the refrigerator for up to 5 days.

Yield: About 4⅓ cups

A good source of: potent antioxidants, chlorophyll, vitamins B and C, potassium, magnesium, sulfur, slow-release carbohydrates, and fiber

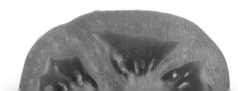

Sweet Banana-Avocado Dip

I know, the pairing of banana with avocado sounds bizarre, but give it a whirl and you'll find the combination utterly luscious, sweet, and creamy. This recipe makes a smashing dip for celery sticks, carrot sticks, whole strawberries, and apple and pear slices. Try a snack featuring this dip after a long workout or an exhausting day of running errands or chasing children.

1 medium, ripe Hass avocado

1 medium, ripe banana

1 tablespoon raw honey

1 tablespoon fresh lemon juice

dash of ground cinnamon

pinch of sea salt

❶ Slice the avocado in half lengthwise, remove the pit, and scoop out the flesh. Peel and cut the banana into rough chunks. Transfer the avocado and banana to a food processor and add the honey, lemon juice, cinnamon, and salt. Blend until smooth and super-creamy, about 30 seconds.

❷ Store the dip in a tightly sealed container in the refrigerator for up to 2 days.

Yield: About 1¼ cups

A good source of: antioxidants plus vitamins B and C, potassium, magnesium, natural sugars, healthful fat, and fiber

Tahini Tango Dip

This is a very basic tahini dip — one of my favorites, as the strong sesame flavor has not been drowned out or diluted by lots of additional herbs and spices. For a fresh snack, I like to spread some on red bell pepper slices or celery sticks.

1 garlic clove, peeled and minced

3 tablespoons fresh lemon juice

1 cup raw tahini

2 tablespoons extra-virgin olive oil

2 tablespoons purified water

½ teaspoon sea salt (add more, if desired)

1 Combine the garlic, lemon juice, tahini, oil, water, and salt in a medium bowl. Whisk vigorously to blend until thick, smooth, and creamy.

2 Store in a tightly sealed container in the refrigerator for up to 1 week. If it separates a bit, simply give it a few quick stirs to recombine.

Yield: About 1½ cups

A good source of: antioxidants, vitamins B and E, calcium, copper, zinc, iron, phosphorus, magnesium, potassium, manganese, healthful fat, protein, and fiber

Vital Vegan Pesto

I relish pesto when I can make it fresh in summer and put a dollop on almost everything. This vegan version is so smooth and luscious that you'll never miss the Parmesan cheese.

2 cups fresh basil leaves, packed

1 cup raw walnuts or pine nuts

¾ cup extra-virgin olive oil

1 garlic clove, peeled and crushed

1–1½ teaspoons sea salt

¼–½ teaspoon freshly ground black pepper

1 Wash the basil. Remove the larger stems and gently pat dry. Place the basil in a colander and allow it to air-dry for 1 hour. You don't want to introduce water into the pesto, as it will cause it to spoil prematurely.

2 Put the basil in a blender first, followed by the nuts, oil, garlic, salt, and pepper. Blend on medium until you achieve a slightly grainy yet relatively smooth consistency, 20 to 30 seconds. If you prefer, a food processor works equally well.

3 Store in a tightly sealed container in the refrigerator no longer than 2 weeks, for maximum freshness and flavor.

Yield: About 1½ cups

A good source of: healthful fat, including antioxidants omega-3 fatty acids, blood-building chlorophyll, potassium, phosphorus, copper, zinc, calcium, iron, magnesium, calcium, manganese, B vitamins, protein, and fiber

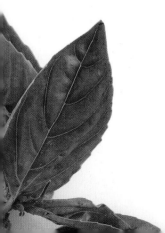

Sweet and Creamy "Cheese" Spread

A nondairy, sweetened "cream cheese" that's out of this world!
I slather this mild, creamy spread on everything — strawberries,
carrot and celery sticks, young asparagus spears, bell pepper
slices, dehydrated cookies, and sprouted Essene bread. I've even
been known to enjoy it straight from the spoon. It has a rich,
slightly figgy-sweet flavor. You must try this recipe!

3 large, dried Calimyrna
  or Turkish figs

1 tablespoon fresh lemon
  juice

1 cup raw cashews

1 tablespoon raw honey

½ teaspoon sea salt

A good source of:
B vitamins, potassium,
calcium, selenium,
magnesium, phosphorus,
iron, copper, zinc,
protein, healthful
fat, slow-release
carbohydrates, and fiber

❶ Soak the figs in a small bowl for 6 hours,
completely covered by purified water. Drain and
reserve ¼ cup of the sweet soak liquid.

❷ Trim the stems from the figs and put the fruit
and reserved soaking liquid in a food processor. Add
the lemon juice, cashews, honey, and salt and blend
until smooth and creamy, 2 to 3 minutes. Scrape the
sides of the food processor with a spatula as needed
to incorporate all of the cashew bits. Expect the
light crunch of fig seeds to remain.

❸ Store in a tightly sealed container in the
refrigerator for up to 1 week.

Yield: About 1¼ cups

Steph's "Big Tex" Guacamole Dip

Texans are huge fans of guacamole and eat it with almost every-thing, including their breakfast tacos. In spite of being heavy on healthful fats, this chunky, zippy dip is very energizing. Regular consumption of guacamole will do wonders to promote a clear, moist, glowing complexion and a shiny head of hair!

2 medium, ripe Hass avocados

1 cup roughly chopped tomatoes

½ cup diced or minced red onion

2 garlic cloves, peeled and crushed

1 medium jalapeño pepper

¼ cup cilantro leaves, tightly packed

¼ cup lime juice

¾ teaspoon sea salt

½ teaspoon freshly ground black pepper

1 Slice the avocados in half lengthwise, remove the pits, and scoop the flesh into a medium bowl. Mash thoroughly with a fork.

2 Stir the tomatoes, onion, and garlic into the mashed avocados.

3 Seed and mince the jalapeño and finely chop the cilantro leaves. Add both to the avocado mixture.

4 Stir in the lime juice and sprinkle salt and pepper over the mixture. Mash everything together with your fork until you achieve a chunky-smooth consistency.

5 Serve immediately, or store in a tightly sealed container in the refrigerator for up to 4 hours.

Yield: About 2½ cups

A good source of: vitamins B and C, antioxidants, sulfur, potassium, magnesium, chlorophyll, protein, slow-release carbohydrates, and fiber

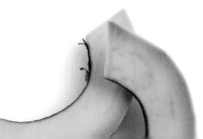

Sunny Vegetable Pâté

This most delectable vegetable pâté is quite hearty in texture, yet not too heavy on the digestive system. It's wonderful used as a dip for crudités, stuffed into small hollowed tomatoes, or as a substantial spread on sprouted Essene bread or flax crackers.

2 tablespoons parsley leaves, packed

1 medium red or orange bell pepper

1 cup raw, hulled sunflower seeds

1 bunch scallions, cut into 1-inch pieces (about ¾ cup)

¼ cup extra-virgin olive oil

1 tablespoon fresh lemon juice

1 tablespoon Bragg Liquid Aminos (raw soy sauce)

½ teaspoon sea salt

½ teaspoon freshly ground black pepper

dash of cayenne pepper

❶ Chop the parsley. Roughly chop the bell pepper, removing the core.

❷ Put the parsley, bell pepper, sunflower seeds, scallions, oil, lemon juice, soy sauce, salt, pepper, and cayenne in a food processor. Blend for 60 to 90 seconds, until thick with a smooth yet granular texture from the tiny vegetable bits.

❸ Store in a tightly sealed container in the refrigerator for up to 5 days.

Yield: About 2 cups

A good source of: antioxidants, vitamins B, C, D, E, and K, zinc, iron, sulfur, potassium, magnesium, manganese, selenium, phosphorus, copper, protein, slow-release carbohydrates, chlorophyll, healthful fat, and fiber

Curried Cashew-Onion Dip

This recipe makes a slightly sweet, rich, creamy, zesty alternative to classic, sour cream-based onion dip. I find it most luscious stuffed into celery ribs or small hollowed tomatoes, or spread on sprouted Essene bread or flax crackers.

1 cup raw cashews

1 medium onion, roughly chopped (about ¾ cup)

3 tablespoons fresh lemon juice

2 tablespoons extra-virgin olive oil

1 tablespoon flaxseed oil

1 teaspoon curry powder

¾ teaspoon sea salt

½ teaspoon freshly ground black pepper

❶ Put the cashews, onion, lemon juice, olive oil, flaxseed oil, curry powder, salt, and pepper in a food processor and blend until smooth, about 3 minutes. Scrape the sides of the food processor with a spatula as needed to incorporate all of the cashew bits into the dip.

❷ Store in a tightly sealed container in the refrigerator for up to 1 week.

Yield: About 1½ cups

A good source of: vitamins B and C, magnesium, calcium, phosphorus, potassium, sulfur, copper, iron, zinc, selenium, plenty of healthful fat, slow-release carbohydrates, protein, and fiber

Basic Fruit Jam

A lip-smacking, vitality-boosting jam recipe made without all the boiling, stirring, and nutritionally empty refined sugar. For instant energy, eat it by the spoonful or mix with a couple of tablespoons of raw nut butter and spread on a banana or celery stalk. It works nicely as a mild sweetener in smoothies and shakes, as a fruit layer in parfaits, and as a topping on muesli.

- ¼ cup roughly chopped dried apples, tightly packed
- ¼ cup roughly chopped unsweetened dried mango, tightly packed
- ¼ cup dried blueberries, sweetened with apple juice, or unsweetened
- ¼ cup raisins
- pinch of sea salt

A good source of:
antioxidants, iron, potassium, boron, magnesium, fiber, and natural sugars

1. Put the apples, mango, blueberries, raisins, and salt in a medium bowl. Add enough purified water to completely cover the mixture by about 1 inch. Soak the mixture on the kitchen counter for 8 to 12 hours or overnight, until the fruits are nice and plump. If the house is hot, cover the bowl and place it in the refrigerator.

2. Drain the excess soak water into a small bowl or cup. Cover and refrigerate. You can enjoy this later as a sweet, refreshing, mineral-rich energizing drink.

3. Put the plumped fruits in a blender or food processor. Pulse-chop or blend on medium until you have a chunky paste resembling thick fruit sauce, 15 to 30 seconds.

4. Store the jam in a tightly sealed container in the refrigerator for up to 2 weeks.

Yield: About 1⅓ cups

Hot and Spicy Zucchini-Scallion Dip

Zucchini and scallions take center stage here for a light-textured, zippy dip. The garlic and cayenne lend a pungent bite, increasing your circulation and stimulating your core metabolism. Perfect as a luscious dip for crudités, stuffing for small hollowed tomatoes, or simply enjoyed by the spoonful.

3 medium zucchini, peeled and cut into chunks (about 2 cups)

1 bunch scallions, cut into 1-inch pieces (about ¾ cup)

½ cup raw tahini

¼ cup extra-virgin olive oil

juice of 1 medium lemon (about ¼ cup)

2 garlic cloves, peeled and crushed

1 teaspoon sea salt or your favorite herbal seasoning salt

¾ teaspoon cayenne pepper (use ¼ teaspoon for a milder "bite")

❶ Put the zucchini, scallions, tahini, oil, lemon juice, garlic, salt, and cayenne in a food processor and blend until thick and creamy, about 60 seconds.

❷ Store in a tightly sealed container in the refrigerator for up to 1 week.

Yield: About 2¼ cups

A good source of: antioxidants, vitamins B, C, and E, calcium, potassium, phosphorus, chlorophyll, magnesium, manganese, copper, zinc, iron, sulfur, protein, healthful fat, and fiber

Chapter 10

CHILLIN'
FRESH, COLD FRUIT AND VEGETABLE SOUPS

TAHITIAN MANGO GINGER SOUP

Tahitian Mango Ginger Soup

This thick, brilliant-orange soup trumpets an exquisite combination of tropical fruit flavors mingled with a delicate hint of warming spices. It's guaranteed to supercharge your vitality and quell your appetite. This soup is also a superior source of digestive enzymes and a fabulous kidney cleanser and mild diuretic, and it helps clear the skin of acne.

3 medium ripe mangoes, peeled and pitted (about 3 cups)

juice of 1 medium orange, tangerine, or tangelo (about ⅓ cup)

¼ cup purified water

2 tablespoons fresh lime juice

1 tablespoon raw honey

1 teaspoon gingerroot, peeled and minced

¼ teaspoon curry powder

¼ teaspoon sea salt

3 mint sprigs (optional, for garnish)

❶ Put the mango, orange juice, water, lime juice, honey, ginger, curry powder, and salt in a blender. Blend on medium until very smooth and relatively thick, about 60 seconds.

❷ For the best flavor, chill the soup for at least 4 hours before serving. Garnish each bowl of soup with a mint sprig, if desired. Store in a tightly sealed container in the refrigerator for up to 48 hours.

Yield: 3 servings

A good source of: antioxidants, potassium, vitamin C, natural sugars, and fiber, and lesser amounts of vitamin K, phosphorus, magnesium, and calcium

Garden Gazpacho

The ultimate summertime cold soup offers refreshment in every spoonful. Gazpacho is best made when the ingredients can be picked fresh from the garden or purchased from the local farmers' market. Using hard, flavorless tomatoes out of season will simply not do!

3 medium tomatoes, roughly chopped (about 3 cups)

1 medium bell pepper, seeded and roughly chopped (about 1 cup)

1 medium cucumber, peeled and roughly chopped

½ cup diced onion

1 garlic clove, peeled and minced

1 tablespoon flaxseed oil

1 teaspoon sea salt

1 teaspoon freshly ground black pepper

1 medium Hass avocado, pitted and diced (optional, for garnish)

❶ Place the tomatoes, bell pepper, cucumber, onion, garlic, flaxseed oil, salt, and pepper in a food processor and pulse-chop until blended to a chunky-soupy consistency. Blending shouldn't take more than 30 seconds.

❷ For the best flavor, chill the soup for at least 4 hours before serving. Garnish each bowl with a handful of diced avocado, if desired. Store in a tightly sealed container in the refrigerator for up to 4 days.

Yield: 4 servings

A good source of: antioxidants, vitamin C, potassium, silicon, sulfur, omega-3 fatty acids, fiber, and hydrating vegetable juices

Honey Melon Pear Soup

Pale, lime green, thick and fruity, and bursting with juicy flavor, this thirst-quenching soup is the height of fruit delight. A small bowlful instantly refreshes and adds zip to your flagging energy stores, especially if it's consumed following a strenuous workout or an afternoon spent harvesting vegetables under the hot summer sun. This soup, if eaten regularly, will help remedy constipation, leaving you feeling like your old self again!

1 medium, very ripe honeydew melon

1 medium, very ripe Packham, Comice, or Bartlett pear, cored and roughly chopped (about 1 cup)

1 tablespoon fresh lime juice

2 teaspoons raw honey

pinch of sea salt

① Cut the melon in half, remove the seeds, and scoop out the flesh, getting as close to the rind as possible. Place the melon in a blender along with the pear, lime juice, honey, and salt. Blend on medium until velvety smooth, about 20 seconds.

② For the best flavor, chill the soup for at least 2 hours before serving. Store in a tightly sealed container in the refrigerator for up to 24 hours. If the soup separates, reblend or stir vigorously for a few seconds.

Yield: 4 servings

A good source of: potassium, plus vitamin C, magnesium, silicon, folic acid, natural sugars, and fiber

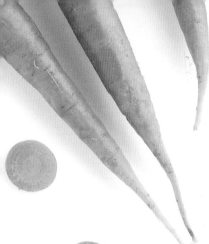

Dreamy Carrot Cream Soup

A delightfully light, gently spicy soup that will increase vitality, beautify your complexion, and add strength and luster to fingernails and hair. Every bowlful of this simple soup offers a bevy of benefits!

2 pounds carrots, juiced (about 2½ cups juice)

1 small sweet onion, such as Vidalia, diced (about ⅓ cup)

1 teaspoon peeled and minced gingerroot

½ cup raw cashews

½ teaspoon sea salt

¼ teaspoon curry powder

1 Put the carrot juice, onion, ginger, cashews, salt, and curry powder in a blender. Blend on medium until relatively smooth, about 60 seconds.

2 For the best flavor, chill the soup for at least 1 hour before serving. Store in a tightly sealed container in the refrigerator for up to 12 hours.

Yield: *3 servings*

A good source of: antioxidants, vitamins B and C, phosphorus, potassium, calcium, magnesium, copper, sulfur, selenium, iron, zinc, protein, natural sugars, and healthful fat

Raspberry Ricky Soup

A stunningly brilliant pinkish red, this soup has a smooth, delicate texture and a refreshing sweet-tart flavor; it's perfect served as a cooling dinnertime appetizer or dessert. When summer is at its steamiest and you're expecting company, blend up a few batches. Raspberry Ricky Soup is one of my favorites, especially when the berries can be picked fresh from the bush!

2½ cups fresh or frozen (thawed) red raspberries

juice of 1 medium lime (about ¼ cup)

¼ cup raw honey

dash of ground cinnamon

pinch of sea salt

2 mint sprigs for garnish (optional, for garnish)

❶ Put the raspberries, lime juice, honey, cinnamon, and salt in a blender and blend on medium until smooth, about 30 seconds. You will see tiny raspberry seeds suspended in the purée.

❷ To remove the seeds, strain the blended liquid through a mesh strainer directly into a storage container.

❸ For the best flavor, chill the soup for at least 2 hours before serving. As a decorative garnish, top each bowl with a fresh mint sprig, if desired. Store in a tightly sealed container in the refrigerator for up to 48 hours.

Yield: 2 servings

A good source of: antioxidants, vitamins B, C, and K, potassium, magnesium, manganese, calcium, natural sugars, and fiber

Cool Cucumber Cress Soup

This wonderfully light, cooling, and refreshing soup offers a bevy of benefits: it's thirst-quenching, complexion-clarifying, stimulating to the circulation, blood-building and purifying, and, because it acts as a gentle diuretic, eliminating excess water and under-eye puffiness, it's also kidney-cleansing.

3 medium cucumbers, peeled and roughly chopped

1 cup watercress, packed, larger stems removed

¼ cup diced onion

½ cup purified water

2 tablespoons fresh lemon juice

2 tablespoons Bragg Liquid Aminos (raw soy sauce)

2 tablespoons flaxseed oil

❶ Put the cucumbers, watercress, onion, water, lemon juice, soy sauce, and flaxseed oil in a blender.

❷ Blend on medium until relatively smooth, about 2 minutes. Expect tiny bits of watercress to remain visible in the finished soup.

❸ For the best flavor, chill the soup for at least 6 hours before serving. The flavors will mellow and lose their initial sharpness. Store in a tightly sealed container in the refrigerator for up to 48 hours.

Yield: 3 servings

A good source of: chlorophyll, antioxidants, vitamins C and K, potassium, silicon, sulfur, iodine, calcium, omega-3 fatty acids, and fiber

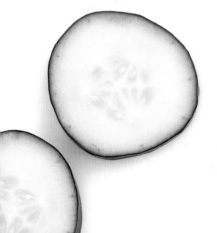

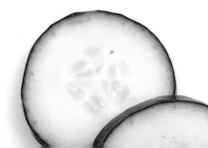

Papaya Sunset Soup

This rich, pinkish orange soup offers a tropical lusciousness that must be experienced. Its taste is reminiscent of fresh apricot nectar spiked with pungent gingerroot juice, mellowed by flavors of vanilla and honey. For athletes and other active people, it serves as a superb — almost instant — thirst-quenching restorative snack following a workout or exhausting hot day spent in the garden or doing heavy landscaping. Consumed regularly, papaya will greatly benefit the condition of the hair, skin, and nails; it can also improve vision.

---

3 medium papayas

⅓ cup purified water

2 tablespoons fresh lime juice

2 tablespoons raw honey

1 teaspoon vanilla extract

¼ teaspoon sea salt

2 large strawberries, sliced (optional garnish)

❶ Slice the papayas in half lengthwise and remove the seeds. Scoop the flesh into a blender and add the water, lime juice, honey, vanilla, and salt. Blend on medium until very smooth, 30 to 45 seconds.

❷ For the best flavor, chill the soup for at least 2 hours before serving. Top each bowl with sliced strawberries, if desired. Store in a tightly sealed container in the refrigerator for up to 48 hours.

Yield: 2 servings

A good source of: digestive enzymes, carotenoids and natural sugars, plus vitamin C, potassium, folic acid, calcium, and fiber

Cucumber Avocado Cream Soup

A pale green, mildly flavored, creamy blend that's filling yet light, with an essence of peppery zing, this soup serves as a perfect afternoon pick-me-up or summertime appetizer when entertaining dinner guests. It is a true "beauty soup" in that the nutrients will encourage your hair, skin, and nails to glow. Cucumber is a natural diuretic, which will aid in draining the body of retained water and related puffiness.

1 medium Hass avocado
1 medium cucumber
1 medium jalapeño pepper
1 tablespoon fresh lemon juice
½ cup purified water
½ teaspoon sea salt
¼ teaspoon freshly ground black or white pepper

❶ Slice the avocado in half lengthwise and remove the pit. Scoop the flesh into a blender. Peel and chop the cucumber; add it to the blender. Slice the jalapeño in half lengthwise, remove and discard the seeds, and mince. Add the jalapeño, lemon juice, water, salt, and pepper to the blender and blend on medium until smooth and creamy, 60 to 90 seconds.

❷ For the best flavor, cover and chill the soup for at least 2 hours before serving, or store in a tightly sealed container in the refrigerator for up to 24 hours.

Yield: 2 small servings

A good source of: antioxidants, B, C, and E vitamins, potassium, magnesium, silicon, protein, slow-release carbohydrates, healthful fat, fiber, and lesser amounts of easily absorbed iron, copper, and calcium

Chapter 11

RAW CONFECTIONS: NO-GUILT, NUTRIENT-PACKED CANDY AND COOKIES

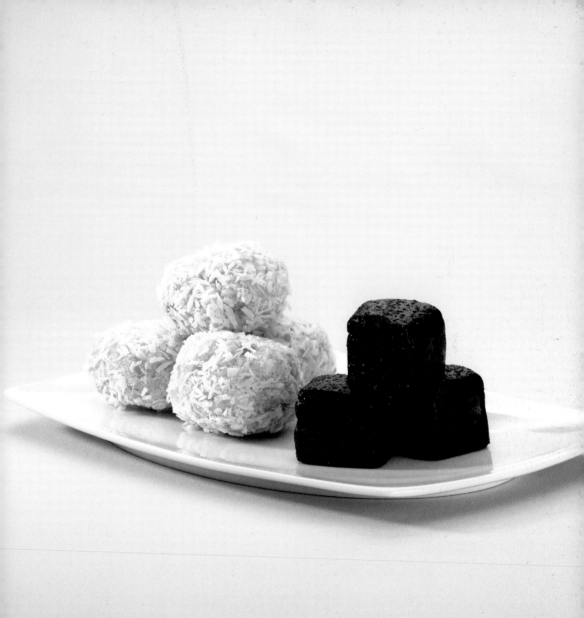

CHEWY APRICOT MACAROONS AND CREAMY CAROB FREEZER FUDGE

I've saved the best and most decadent yummies for the last chapter. This section is filled with recipes for indulgent sweet treats that will satisfy that ever-present craving for all things sticky, gooey, fruity, sinful, fudgy, and chocolaty . . . all without a smidgen of refined, empty-calorie ingredients such as sugar, white flour, corn syrup, artificial color, fake fruit bits, synthetic flavoring, and marshmallow creme.

These candies, cookies, and fudge treats are made from a mix of wholesome nuts, seeds, and butters, dried fruits, oats, honey, agave nectar, maple syrup, raw cocoa (cacao), carob, coconut, spices and flavorings, all blended together to yield delicious raw confections that will help boost your energy while healthfully satisfying a raging sweet tooth. I believe you'll be amazed at the variety of recipes offered. There's something for everyone — even the most finicky.

A plateful of any of these goodies makes a terrific dessert for both casual family events and formal dinner affairs. I hope you enjoy making (and eating) these luscious sweets as much as I do. I guarantee that after you've tasted your first bite of raw fudge and discovered how easy it is to make, you'll never go back to its refined, sugary, cooked cousin again!

Stuffed Date Bites

This deliciously simple snack is a mighty morsel of portable energy. It combines the intense sweetness of dates with the creaminess of pecans. Wrap these bites in waxed paper or plastic wrap and take them with you to serve as portable energy treats. Consider it a nice tidy package with nutritional punch!

12 Medjool or your favorite moist, large dates

12 large raw pecans

1 Slice each date lengthwise and remove the pit. Insert a pecan into the center of the date and press to seal closed so you have a date-pecan sandwich.

2 For the best flavor, store the bites in a tightly sealed container in the refrigerator for no more than 4 weeks or at room temperature for no more than 2 weeks.

Yield: 12 servings

A good source of: antioxidants, calcium, magnesium, phosphorus, iron, zinc, copper, manganese, potassium, protein, vitamin B and E, natural sugars, fiber, and healthful fat

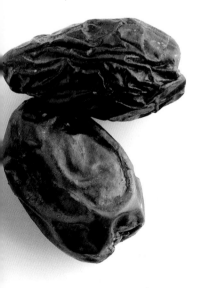

Carob Halvah

Halvah is a traditional Middle Eastern sesame candy that's not too sweet and is slightly dry and chewy. My recipe gives traditional halvah a delectable carob twist that I'm sure you'll savor. These candies can be individually wrapped in plastic wrap or waxed paper, and packed in your purse, gym bag, briefcase, or backpack — just don't let them get too warm and soft. Pop a couple of these candies anytime you're in need of a sweet bite and a bit of vigor. Eat these goodies often enough and your hair, skin, and nails will glow with strength.

1 cup raw sesame seeds, hulled or unhulled

1 tablespoon raw carob powder

dash of ground cinnamon

pinch of sea salt

¼ cup raw honey

2 tablespoons raw tahini

1 teaspoon vanilla extract

❶ Put the sesame seeds in a food processor and blend until you achieve a medium-coarse meal, 60 to 90 seconds. Transfer the seed meal to a large bowl.

❷ Add the carob, cinnamon, and salt to the sesame seeds and blend well with a large spoon or whisk.

❸ Drizzle the honey, tahini, and vanilla over the dry mix. If the honey is thick and stiff, set the container in a pan of hot water for a few minutes to thin it.

❹ Using your hands, mash and knead the ingredients until a cohesive, granular, stiff dough ball forms.

5 Pull off bits of dough and form into balls about 1 inch in diameter.

6 Store the halvah in the refrigerator in a tightly sealed container for up to 3 weeks or in the freezer for up to 6 months. It can be enjoyed right out of the freezer.

Yield: About 22 candies

A good source of: vitamins B and E, calcium, magnesium, iron, potassium, copper, zinc, phosphorus, manganese, protein, natural sugars, healthful fat, and fiber

Fabulous Coco-Walnut Fudgy Brownies

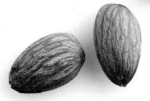

Not only are these brownies fabulously flavorful, but they're fabulous for your health to boot! Individually wrap them or carry them in a small container — just don't let them get too warm or they'll become very soft. If you just have to have a bite of energizing chocolate, this hearty, sweet combination satisfies on all levels.

8	Medjool dates, pitted
1½	cups raw walnuts
1	cup raw oat flakes
½	cup raw almond butter
½	cup raw cocoa (cacao) powder
	dash of ground cinnamon
	pinch of sea salt
	coconut oil, raw and unrefined (for greasing pan)

❶ Soak the dates for 3 hours in enough purified water to cover by 1 inch. Drain and reserve the soak water, if desired. It can be sipped chilled or used to sweeten a smoothie.

❷ Blend the walnuts in a food processor to a moist, semicoarse meal, 20 to 30 seconds.

❸ Add the dates, oats, almond butter, cocoa, cinnamon, and salt to the food processor and blend until a cohesive, moist-but-not-sticky dough forms, about 30 seconds.

❹ Oil an 8-inch square pan with coconut oil. Using your hands or a spatula, press the dough into the pan to a thickness of about ¾ inch.

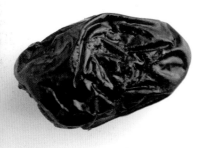

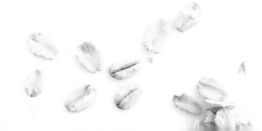

5 Place the covered pan in the freezer for 2 hours. Remove and cut the brownies into 1½-inch squares. Store in a tightly sealed container in the freezer for up to 3 months or in the refrigerator for up to 2 weeks.

Yield: About 24 brownies

A good source of: antioxidants, vitamins B and E, calcium, phosphorus, potassium, sulfur, copper, selenium, manganese, magnesium, iron, zinc, omega-3 fatty acids, protein, natural sugars, slow-release carbohydrates, and fiber, plus a touch of caffeine (from the cocoa) that gently stimulates circulation

Creamy Carob Freezer Fudge

Not too sweet but rich, dark, and velvety, this is the ultimate in decadent creamy, melt-in-your-mouth, smoothly textured fudge. Right out of the freezer, it's a great warm-weather treat that provides plenty of energy to keep your metabolism running at peak performance.

12 Medjool dates, pitted
1 cup raw almond butter
1 cup raw carob powder
2 tablespoons raw honey
    dash of grated nutmeg
    pinch of sea salt
    coconut oil, raw and unrefined (for greasing pan)

A good source of: vitamins B and E, calcium, magnesium, manganese, potassium, phosphorus, iron, zinc, protein, natural sugars, healthful fat, and fiber

❶ Soak the dates for 4 hours in enough purified water to cover by 1 inch. Drain and reserve the soak water, if desired. It can be sipped chilled or used to sweeten a smoothie.

❷ Put the dates, almond butter, carob, honey, nutmeg, and salt in a food processor and blend until a cohesive, moist, almost elastic dough forms, 20 to 30 seconds.

❸ Oil an 8-inch square pan with coconut oil. Using your hands or a spatula, press the dough into the pan to a thickness of about ¾ inch.

❹ Place the covered pan in the freezer for 4 hours to harden the fudge prior to cutting. Remove the pan and cut the fudge into 1½-inch squares. Store in a tightly sealed container in the freezer for up to 3 months. Do not store in the refrigerator; it will become too soft.

Yield: About 24 squares

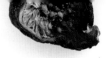

Sesame Calcium Chews

Regular consumption of this mildly sweet, raw candy will lend a glow to your hair, skin, and nails, replenish your core energy reserve, or ojas, and strengthen your bones.

20 small, dried, Black Mission figs

1 cup raw sesame seeds, hulled or unhulled

2 tablespoons raw honey

pinch of sea salt

½ cup unsweetened coconut, finely shredded

A good source of:
vitamins B and E,
iron, copper, zinc,
magnesium, calcium,
phosphorus, potassium,
manganese, natural
sugars, protein,
healthful fat, and fiber

❶ Remove the stems from the figs. Soak the figs for 4 hours in enough purified water to cover by 1 inch. Drain. Reserve the chilled soak water to drink later for a refreshing treat.

❷ Put the figs, sesame seeds, honey, and salt in a food processor and blend for 20 to 30 seconds. Remove the lid and scrape down the sides of the bowl with a spatula. Replace the lid and blend again until a moist, slightly sticky, granular dough forms, about 10 seconds.

❸ Scrape the dough into a medium bowl. Put the coconut in another medium bowl.

❹ Pinch off pieces of the dough and roll into balls approximately 1 inch in diameter. Toss the balls in the coconut to coat.

❺ Store in a tightly sealed container in the refrigerator for up to 3 weeks or in the freezer for up to 6 months. The chews are delicious eaten right out of the freezer.

Yield: 25 to 30 balls

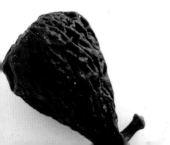

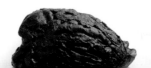

Chewy Apricot Macaroons

If you're a fan of coconut and apricots, you'll love these fruity, sweet macaroons. This is the perfect treat to restore your vigor following a strenuous day of work or play.

1½ cups dried apricots

3 cups unsweetened coconut, finely shredded

pinch of sea salt

❶ Soak the apricots for 4 hours in enough purified water to cover by 2 inches. Apricots really swell when soaked, so give them ample water and room to expand. Drain thoroughly. Reserve and chill the soak water; it makes a luscious, energizing, very sweet drink.

❷ Blend the apricots, coconut, and salt in a food processor until a stiff, moist, cohesive dough forms, about 60 seconds. If necessary, scrape down the sides of the bowl with a spatula every 15 seconds or so to completely incorporate the coconut.

❸ Scrape the dough into a medium bowl. Using your hands, roll the dough into balls about 1½ inches in diameter and flatten slightly to form a mounded cookie shape. Place the macaroons on mesh dehydrator screens and dehydrate at 115°F (46°C) for 18 to 22 hours, until quite firm and slightly crispy on the outside and chewy on the inside.

❹ When drying is complete, remove the screens from the dehydrator and allow the cookies to cool for 20 minutes.

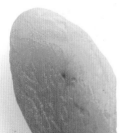

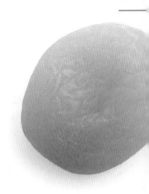

5 Store in a tightly sealed container at room temperature for up to 2 weeks or refrigerate for up to 1 month. The initial crispiness will dissipate with storage.

Yield: About 40 cookies

A good source of: antioxidants, plus B vitamins, potassium, phosphorus, calcium, iron, natural sugars, healthful fat, protein, and fiber

Date Logs

Need instant energy? These little date candies are just what the doctor ordered! They'll satisfy your sweet tooth and stave off junk food cravings, too, making a perfect quick snack bite to replenish lost minerals following a workout. Date Logs are just the kind of snack I like: no kitchen appliances required; a little simple mashing and kneading and you're done!

15 Medjool dates, pitted

1 cup unsweetened coconut, finely shredded

½ teaspoon ground cinnamon

pinch of sea salt

A good source of: natural pick-me-up sugars plus B vitamins, potassium, phosphorus, magnesium, iron, healthful fat, protein, and fiber

❶ Soak the dates for 4 hours in enough purified water to cover by 1 inch. Drain and reserve the soak water, if desired. It can be sipped chilled or used to sweeten a smoothie recipe.

❷ Put the dates, coconut, cinnamon, and salt in a large bowl. Using your hands, mash and knead the ingredients until the coconut is incorporated into the mass of moist dates and a stiff dough ball forms.

❸ Pinch off pieces of the dough and roll into nuggets or logs about 2 inches long and 1 inch in diameter.

❹ Store Date Logs in a tightly sealed container in the refrigerator for up to 2 weeks or in the freezer for up to 3 months. They can be eaten right out of the freezer, as they will not become too hard — just very firm.

Yield: About 15 logs

Prune Poppers

Have you eaten a fresh, moist prune lately? If not, you're in for a sweet treat of the energetic kind! Prune Poppers are potent, tasty bites that you can pop in your mouth whenever you need a little lift. These sweets travel well and can be individually wrapped, using waxed paper or plastic wrap, and stashed away in your desk, purse, backpack, or briefcase until a burst of energy is needed. Regular consumption of these snacks will help ease the discomfort of constipation while increasing your intake of vital nutrients and putting a zip back in your step.

12 large, relatively moist prunes

12 raw almonds

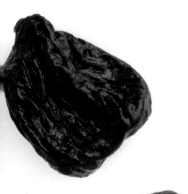

❶ Slice each prune lengthwise and remove the pit, if necessary. Insert an almond into the center of each prune and press to seal closed.

❷ For the best flavor, store the poppers in a tightly sealed container in the refrigerator for no more than 4 weeks or at room temperature for no more than 2 weeks.

Yield: 12 pieces

A good source of: antioxidants, plus plenty of vitamins B and E, iron, zinc, potassium, calcium, magnesium, manganese, phosphorus, natural sugars, protein, healthful fat, and fiber

Chocolate Turtles

Chocolate turtles are a classic confection loved by everyone. This raw, melt-in-your-mouth version is a guilt-free treat when eaten with a glass of cold, fresh almond or walnut milk.

½ cup raw almond butter

½ cup raw cocoa (cacao) powder

¼ cup raw agave nectar

16 small or medium raw pecan halves (about ⅓ cup)

A good source of: antioxidants, plus vitamins B and E, calcium, potassium, phosphorus, sulfur, magnesium, manganese, copper, zinc, iron, natural sugars, protein, healthful fat, and fiber

❶ Put the almond butter, cocoa, and agave in a large bowl and slowly stir to blend until a sticky, stiff dough forms.

❷ Line the bottom of an 8-inch square pan with parchment or waxed paper.

❸ Pinch off pieces of the dough and roll into balls about 1¼ inches in diameter. Rinse and dry your hands periodically if they get too sticky. Set the balls into the pan so they are not touching.

❹ Gently press a pecan half into the top of each ball. Cover the pan and chill in the refrigerator for at least 4 hours prior to consuming. They'll become a little bit firmer but will still be pleasantly soft and chewy. I prefer to store and eat them directly out of the freezer, as they become quite firm but still chewy, and the pecan gets crunchy. Whichever method you choose, always store your candies in a tightly sealed container, either in the refrigerator for up to 3 weeks or in the freezer for up to 3 months.

Yield: About 16 pieces

Vanilla-Walnut "Shortbread" Cookies

These goodies are ultrarich with a melt-in-your-mouth velvety texture bursting with creamy vanilla flavor; they taste a bit like traditional baked shortbread. The dough would make a terrific crust for a raw pie.

2 cups raw walnuts

1 cup unsweetened coconut, finely shredded

¼ cup raw honey

1 teaspoon vanilla extract

pinch of sea salt

❶ Blend the walnuts, coconut, honey, vanilla, and salt in a food processor until a granular, moist dough forms, about 60 seconds. It will not form a cohesive ball and will be very oily when handled.

❷ Scrape the dough into a medium bowl. Pinch off pieces of the dough and gently squeeze, knead, and roll the pieces into balls about 1½ inches in diameter. Press each ball between your palms to slightly flatten into cookies.

❸ Store in a tightly sealed container in the refrigerator for up to 3 weeks or in the freezer for up to 3 months.

Yield: About 22 cookies

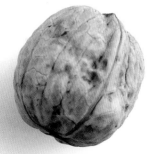

A good source of: omega-3 fatty acids plus B vitamins, calcium, zinc, copper, iron, magnesium, potassium, phosphorus, manganese, natural sugars, protein, and fiber — all of which provide for a constant flow of energy

Cashew Clusters

This mildly flavored but slightly crunchy snack satisfies your sweet tooth while providing an energetic lift with real staying power. No empty calories here!

12 Medjool dates, pitted
1½ cups raw cashews
½ teaspoon vanilla extract
dash of ground nutmeg or cardamom
pinch of sea salt

A good source of:

B vitamins, potassium, selenium, phosphorus, magnesium, iron, zinc, copper, healthful fat, natural sugars, protein, and fiber

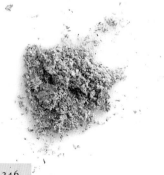

❶ Soak the dates for 4 hours in enough purified water to cover by 1 inch. Drain and reserve the soak water, if desired. It can be added to sweeten a smoothie recipe or sipped chilled.

❷ Grind the cashews in a food processor until they are coarsely chopped and chunky, about 10 seconds. Do not grind the nuts into a coarse meal. Pour the cashews into a medium bowl.

❸ Add the dates, vanilla, nutmeg, and salt to the food processor and blend into a semi-granular paste, about 10 seconds. Scrape the paste into the bowl of chopped cashews.

❹ Using the back of a large spoon or your hands, mash and knead the ingredients until a chunky, cohesive dough ball forms.

❺ Pinch off pieces of the dough and roll into balls about 1¼ inches in diameter. If your hands become too sticky, rinse with warm water, dry, and begin rolling again.

❻ Store the nut clusters in a tightly sealed container in the refrigerator for up to 2 weeks.

Yield: About 20 clusters

Hazelnut Heavens

These chewy, slightly crumbly treats offer a sweet and nutty flavor that is indeed heavenly, especially when combined with the tang of dried cherries. They are wonderful when munched for a quick, energy-boosting breakfast or afternoon snack accompanied by a fresh cold glass of almond milk or fresh-squeezed tangerine juice. Yum!

1 cup raw hazelnuts

½ cup dried, pitted cherries, sweetened with apple juice or unsweetened

½ cup raw tahini

3 tablespoons raw honey

dash of ground cinnamon

pinch of sea salt

A good source of:
antioxidants, vitamins B and E, calcium, potassium, magnesium, manganese, phosphorus, iron, zinc, silicon, copper, protein, healthful fat, natural sugars, and fiber

❶ Put the hazelnuts, cherries, tahini, honey, cinnamon, and salt in a food processor and blend for 20 seconds. Scrape down the sides of the bowl with a spatula and blend again for about 60 seconds, until a granular, moist mixture forms.

❷ Scrape the mixture into a medium bowl. Scoop out 1 tablespoon of the mixture and roll and squeeze it in the palm of your hand until it sticks together. Expect the mixture to be quite oily. Gently form into a ball about 1¼ inches in diameter. Repeat procedure with the remainder of the mixture.

❸ For the best flavor and texture, chill the balls for at least 4 hours prior to eating. Store in a tightly sealed container in the refrigerator for up to 2 weeks or in the freezer for up to 2 months.

Yield: About 25 balls

Mexican Dark Chocolate-Blueberry Divine Fudge

Experience raw candy decadence at its finest! If you're familiar with the taste of Mexican chocolate, then you know it can have a pungent bite. This unique fudge has plenty of tongue-tantalizing flavors and textures: bitter and sweet, hot and rich, smooth and chewy, melt-in-your-mouth gooey! With regular consumption, you'll see an increase in outer glow and feel a surge of inner vitality from this luscious, nutrient-packed confection.

½ cup raw, unrefined coconut oil

1 cup dried blueberries, sweetened with apple juice, or unsweetened

1 cup raw cocoa (cacao) powder

½ cup raw almond butter

2 tablespoons raw agave nectar

1 teaspoon chili powder

1 teaspoon ground cinnamon

½ teaspoon cayenne pepper

¼ teaspoon sea salt

❶ If the coconut oil is solid, set the jar in a pan of very hot water or in a warm sunny window to liquefy.

❷ Put the coconut oil, blueberries, cocoa, almond butter, agave, chili powder, cinnamon, cayenne, and salt in a large bowl and stir to blend until a stiff ball forms; there will be small lumps of blueberries.

❸ Coat the bottom of an 8-inch square pan with coconut oil or line with waxed paper. Spread the fudge mixture into the pan to an approximate depth of 1 inch. Cover and freeze for 1 hour, until very firm.

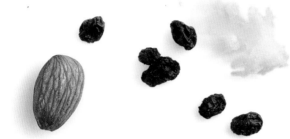

④ Remove from the freezer and allow the mixture to soften slightly for about 20 minutes. Cut the fudge into 1½-inch squares. Store in a tightly sealed container in the refrigerator for up to 2 months or in the freezer for 6 months. Do not allow the fudge to sit at room temperature for too long or it will melt.

Yield: About 24 pieces

A good source of: antioxidants, vitamins B and E, calcium, sulfur, magnesium, potassium, phosphorus, zinc, copper, manganese, iron, natural sugars, healthful fat, protein, and fiber

Easy Peanut Butter and Honey Raisin Fudge Balls

A dream snack for peanut butter and chocolate lovers, these balls will take the edge off a raging sweet tooth and appetite plus help to maintain vital energy stores. This recipe is not totally raw, due to the inclusion of peanut butter, but these fudge balls are simple, hearty, and perfect for young children to make for themselves. They are also great as hiking or travel treats; wrap individually with plastic wrap or waxed paper for easy transportation.

¼ cup raw cocoa (cacao) powder

1 cup natural roasted peanut butter

1 cup small raisins or currants

3 tablespoons raw honey

A good source of: antioxidants, B vitamins, iron, zinc, boron, magnesium, sulfur, manganese, phosphorus, potassium, calcium, copper, natural sugars, protein, healthful fat, and fiber

❶ Put 2 tablespoons of the cocoa in a small bowl and set aside.

❷ Put the remaining 2 tablespoons cocoa, the peanut butter, raisins, and honey in a medium bowl and stir until a stiff dough forms, mixing just to the point that the raisins are incorporated. The dough should appear as a swirly blend of light and dark brown.

❸ Pinch off pieces of the dough and roll into balls about 1 inch in diameter. If your hands become too sticky, rinse in warm water, dry completely, and start rolling again. Gently roll each ball in the bowl of cocoa powder to coat.

❹ Store in a tightly sealed container in the refrigerator for up to 3 weeks or in the freezer for up to 2 months.

Yield: About 36 balls

Almond Coconut Cookies

These unique treats will delight almond lovers with their intense almond flavor and aroma. They're packed with energizing nutrients and make terrific, guilt-free breakfast cookies or anytime pick-me-up snacks. They are also very pretty and look especially tempting arranged on a healthful holiday dessert tray.

2 cups raw almonds

1 cup raw almond butter

3 tablespoons unsweetened coconut, finely shredded.

3 tablespoons raw honey

¼ teaspoon sea salt

¼ teaspoon almond extract

5 or 6 Medjool dates, pitted

A good source of: vitamins B and E, potassium, calcium, magnesium, phosphorus, manganese, zinc, iron, copper, natural sugars, protein, healthful fat, and fiber

❶ Blend the almonds in a food processor until coarsely chopped, about 15 seconds.

❷ Transfer the chopped almonds to a large bowl and blend in the almond butter, coconut, honey, salt, and almond extract. Stir until a stiff, very chunky dough forms. Use your hands to thoroughly blend the ingredients; they will be more effective than a spoon.

❸ Pinch off a piece of the dough about the size of a small walnut and roll between your palms to form a ball that is about 1½ inches in diameter. Gently press the ball between your palms to form a ½-inch-thick cookie. Rinse and dry hands periodically if they become too sticky to roll the balls.

❹ Slice the dates lengthwise and cut the halves into slivers about ⅓ inch wide by 1 inch long. Lightly press a sliver into the center of each cookie for decoration.

❺ Store the cookies in a tightly sealed container in the refrigerator for 2 to 3 weeks.

Yield: About 32 cookies

Cherry-Carob Marbles

Carob and dried cherries make a luscious combo. I adore these ultrasmooth, tasty little bites of power with a glass of fresh almond milk. Pop a couple in your mouth to recharge your energy stores, and you're off and running!

1 cup raw almond butter

¾ cup dried, pitted cherries, sweetened with apple juice or unsweetened

½ cup raw carob powder

¼ cup raw agave nectar

pinch of sea salt

❶ Combine the almond butter, cherries, carob, agave, and salt in a large bowl. Stir well to blend until a stiff dough forms.

❷ Pinch off pieces of the dough and roll into balls about 1 inch in diameter or slightly smaller, if you wish.

❸ Store the balls in a tightly sealed container in the refrigerator for 2 to 3 weeks or in the freezer for up to 3 months. They become quite soft if left at room temperature for too long.

Yield: About 48 bites

A good source of: antioxidants, B and E vitamins, iron, zinc, calcium, potassium, phosphorus, magnesium, manganese, silicon, natural sugars, protein, healthful fat, and fiber

Vegan Dark Chocolate Bliss Pudding

This amazing, fudgy confection should be eaten slowly and savored, one spoonful at a time. It's also absolutely delicious when spread on strawberries, bananas, pear slices, or mixed with raw almond butter. This dairy-free pudding is the perfect treat for hard-core, energy-burning athletes. The rest of us can enjoy it as an occasional indulgent dessert.

½ cup raw, unrefined coconut oil

1 cup raw cocoa (cacao) powder

¾ cup raw honey

dash of ground cinnamon

pinch of sea salt

A good source of: antioxidants, plenty of B vitamins, potassium, calcium, magnesium, manganese, phosphorus, zinc, iron, copper, sulfur, natural sugars, protein, healthful fat, and fiber

❶ If the coconut oil is solid, set the jar in a pan of very hot water or in a warm sunny window to liquefy.

❷ Put the coconut oil, cocoa, honey, cinnamon, and salt in a large bowl and stir rapidly using a spoon or whisk, until very smooth and quite thick, 1 to 2 minutes.

❸ Scrape out the pudding and serve immediately or store in a small, tightly sealed container in the refrigerator for up to 3 weeks. If chilled, it will become very firm and fudgelike. I love to scoop it out of the bowl with a spoon and eat it like this — firm and chewy! To soften it, leave covered at room temperature for 2 or 3 hours.

Yield: 7 servings

Lemon Doodles

The contrasting flavors of sweet buttery richness and light lemony tartness make an invigorating combination. Be careful not to eat too many of these confections; they're addictive! Kids love them, and they make fabulous "finger food" sweets for parties.

4 teaspoons lemon zest (from 2 medium lemons)

2 tablespoons fresh lemon juice

1 cup raw walnuts

½ cup raw sesame seeds, hulled or unhulled

2 tablespoons raw agave nectar

pinch of sea salt

⅓ cup unsweetened coconut, finely shredded

A good source of: vitamins B, C, and E, calcium, potassium, phosphorus, magnesium, manganese, copper, iron, zinc, natural sugars, omega-3 fatty acids, protein, and fiber

❶ Zest the lemons before juicing one lemon for your 2 tablespoons of juice. The other lemon will keep for a few days in the refrigerator for another use.

❷ Put the lemon zest, juice, walnuts, sesame seeds, agave, and salt in a food processor and blend for about 10 seconds. Scrape the mixture from the sides of the bowl with a spatula and blend again for 15 seconds. Repeat once more until a moist, seedy dough ball forms.

❸ Scrape the dough into a medium bowl. Place the coconut in a separate, smaller bowl.

❹ Pinch off pieces of the dough and roll into balls about 1 inch in diameter. Toss the balls in coconut shreds to coat. If your hands get too sticky, wash with warm water, dry, and begin rolling balls again.

❺ Store in a tightly sealed container in the refrigerator for up to 1 week or in the freezer for up to 2 months.

Yield: About 25 treats

Cocoa Snowballs

Crazy for dark chocolate and coconut? These chocolate macaroon balls will surely satisfy! They are simple to make, unbelievably nutritious, rich, and flavorful — and they will satisfy your chocolate craving!

1 vanilla bean, about 7 inches long

1 cup unsweetened coconut, finely shredded

½ cup raw cocoa (cacao) powder

¼ cup coconut oil, raw and unrefined

3 tablespoons raw honey

pinch of sea salt

A good source of:
antioxidants, B vitamins, calcium, iron, phosphorus, magnesium, potassium, zinc, copper, sulfur, manganese, natural sugars, protein, healthful fat, and fiber

❶ Slice the vanilla bean lengthwise and scrape out the seed paste with the tip of a knife. Keep the paste for this recipe and save the remainder of the bean for use in other recipes.

❷ Put the vanilla, coconut, cocoa, coconut oil, honey, and salt in a medium bowl and stir well to blend, making sure that the vanilla bean paste and cocoa powder are thoroughly incorporated. The dough should be relatively stiff.

❸ Pinch off pieces of the dough and roll into balls about 1 inch in diameter.

❹ For the best flavor and texture, chill the balls for at least 4 hours prior to eating. They will be quite firm, but not too hard to easily bite into. Store in a tightly sealed container in the refrigerator for up to 4 weeks.

Yield: About 22 balls

Carob Tangerine Soft and Fudgy Chews

Raw carob candy is amazing! Who would imagine that these chewy, gooey confections could be so full of strength-building goodness with nary a refined, empty ingredient? Due to their high calcium content, regular consumption of these candies will strengthen nails, hair, and bones, and also help relieve muscle cramping, restless legs, and premenstrual syndrome.

zest from 2 medium tangerines, oranges, or tangelos (about 2 tablespoons)

3 tablespoons fresh tangerine, orange, or tangelo juice

1 cup raw carob powder

¾ cup raw tahini

2 tablespoons raw honey

pinch of sea salt

coconut oil, raw and unrefined (for greasing pan)

❶ Zest both pieces of citrus fruit before juicing one piece for your 3 tablespoons of juice. The other fruit will keep for a few days in the refrigerator for another use.

❷ Put the zest, juice, carob, tahini, honey, and salt in a large bowl and stir well, until a relatively stiff dough ball forms. Use your hands to mash and knead the dough if you like.

❸ Grease an 8-inch square pan with coconut oil. Using your hands or a spatula, press the dough into the pan to an even thickness of about ½ inch.

❹ Place the covered pan in the freezer for at least 2 hours. Remove the pan and cut the fudge chews into 1½-inch squares.

5 Store the squares in a tightly sealed container in the freezer for up to 2 months. They will become very gooey and soft if allowed to thaw but will remain chewy and only slightly soft if kept in the freezer.

Yield: About 24 squares

A good source of: vitamins B, C, and E, copper, zinc, iron, calcium, magnesium, manganese, potassium, phosphorus, protein, natural sugars, healthful fat, and fiber

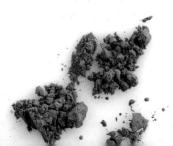

Pecan Raisin Balls

Unbelievably sweet and gooey yet quite rich in natural vitality-building nutrients, these treats will please pecan lovers. I make this simple snack recipe often and enjoy a few bites whenever I need an energizing boost with real staying power.

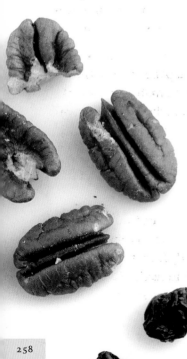

2 cups raw pecans

1 cup small raisins or currants

¼ cup raw agave nectar

pinch of sea salt

❶ Blend the pecans, raisins, agave, and salt in a food processor for 60 to 90 seconds, or until a cohesive dough forms. Expect an oily, soft texture. Scrape the dough into a medium bowl.

❷ Pinch off pieces of the dough and roll into balls about 1 inch in diameter. Your hands will get quite oily and slippery when making the balls; when they do, simply wash with warm water, dry thoroughly, and begin rolling balls again. Repeat as often as necessary.

❸ Store the balls in the refrigerator for up to 2 weeks or in the freezer for up to 2 months.

Yield: About 42 balls

A good source of: antioxidants, vitamins B and E, iron, boron, potassium, magnesium, manganese, phosphorus, zinc, copper, natural sugars, healthful fat, and fiber

Cashew Maple Oatmeal Squares

These sticky and chewy treats will remind you of chilled oatmeal cookie dough. Maple syrup — one of the sweeteners in the recipe — is not raw, but if its scrumptious flavor will encourage your friends and family to eat more raw snacks, then why not use it on occasion? Children will especially love this recipe and benefit from the sustained energy these goodies provide.

10 Medjool dates, pitted and chopped (about 1 cup)

1 cup raw cashews

½ cup raw oats

¼ cup maple syrup

¼ teaspoon ground cinnamon

pinch of sea salt

coconut oil, raw and unrefined (for greasing pan)

A good source of: B vitamins, potassium, phosphorus, selenium, calcium, magnesium, manganese, iron, zinc, copper, slow-release carbohydrates, protein, healthful fat, and fiber

❶ Put the dates, cashews, oats, syrup, cinnamon, and salt in a food processor. Blend until a cohesive, sticky cookie dough forms, about 30 seconds. It will look and taste similar to oatmeal cookie dough.

❸ Coat the bottom of an 8-inch square pan with coconut oil or line with waxed paper. Spread the mixture in the pan to an approximate thickness of ½ inch. If your fingers get too sticky, dampen them to help pat the dough into the pan.

❹ Cover and freeze for 4 hours, until the dough is relatively firm. Remove from the freezer and cut into 1½-inch squares.

❺ Store the squares in a tightly sealed container in the freezer for up to 2 months. They will have a nice, stiff "chew" when eaten directly from the freezer, so don't worry about breaking your teeth. If allowed to thaw, they will become too soft and sticky.

Yield: About 24 squares

Peanut Butter Halvah

A real stick-to-your-ribs, "almost raw" candy that kids adore. Each bite delivers a delightful mélange of flavors that perk up the taste buds. The candy is reminiscent of a peanut butter and honey sandwich with lots of crunch.

1 cup raw oatmeal flakes

1 cup raw sesame seeds, hulled or unhulled

¾ cup natural roasted peanut butter

½ cup raw honey

1 teaspoon vanilla extract

pinch of sea salt

❶ Put the oats, sesame seeds, peanut butter, honey, vanilla, and salt in a large bowl and stir well, until a very stiff dough forms.

❷ Pinch off pieces of the dough and roll into balls about 1 inch in diameter. Your hands will get quite sticky, so when they do, rinse with warm water, dry thoroughly, and resume making balls. Repeat as necessary.

❸ Store the candy in a tightly sealed container in the refrigerator for up to 2 weeks or in the freezer for up to 2 months.

Yield: About 48 balls

A good source of: antioxidants, B and E vitamins, calcium, potassium, selenium, magnesium, iron, phosphorus, copper, zinc, manganese, slow-release carbohydrates, natural sugars, protein, healthful fat, and fiber

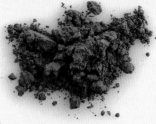

Raw Dark-Chocolate Syrup

Chocolate syrup that's actually good for you? This one is! Because this syrup is free of refined sugar and sweetened with raw agave nectar, which rates low on the glycemic index, it is even suitable for diabetics. My favorite way to enjoy this shiny, decadent syrup is to drizzle it over fresh pear or banana slices, use it as a dip for sweet, ripe strawberries, or drizzle it atop muesli or parfait recipes.

3 tablespoons raw agave nectar

2 tablespoons raw cocoa (cacao) powder

½ teaspoon raw, unrefined coconut oil

⅛ teaspoon vanilla extract

dash of ground cinnamon

pinch of sea salt

1. Put the agave, cocoa, coconut oil, vanilla, cinnamon, and salt in a small bowl and stir vigorously to blend. The mixture should resemble traditional chocolate syrup.

2. Store the syrup in a tightly sealed container and refrigerate for up to 1 month.

Yield: About ⅓ cup

A good source of:
antioxidants, B vitamins, magnesium, calcium, iron, sulfur, phosphorus, potassium, zinc, copper, protein, manganese, fiber, and healthful fat

Suggested Reading

This list contains resources for this book, as well as selections from my personal library that you might find particularly interesting and educational.

Allen, Zel. *The Nut Gourmet: Nourishing Nuts for Every Occasion.* Summertown, TN: Book Publishing Company, 2006.

Alt, Carol. *Eating in the Raw: A Beginner's Guide to Getting Slimmer, Feeling Healthier, and Looking Younger the Raw-Food Way.* New York: Clarkson Potter, 2004.

————. *The Raw 50: 10 Amazing Breakfasts, Lunches, Dinners, Snacks, and Drinks for Your Raw Food Lifestyle.* New York: Clarkson Potter, 2007.

Amsden, Matt. *RAWvolution: Gourmet Living Cuisine.* New York: HarperCollins, 2006.

Balch, Phyllis A. *Prescription for Dietary Wellness,* second edition. New York: Avery, 2003.

Blauer, Stephen. *The Juicing Book: A Complete Guide to the Juicing of Fruits and Vegetables for Maximum Health and Vitality.* New York: Avery, 1989.

Bowden, Jonny. *The 150 Healthiest Foods on Earth: The Surprising, Unbiased Truth About What You Should Eat and Why.* Gloucester, MA: Fair Winds Press, 2007.

Brotman, Juliano, with Erika Lenkert. *RAW: The UNcook Book.* New York: HarperCollins Publishers, 1999.

Cohen, Alissa. *Living on Live Food,* third edition. Kittery, ME: Cohen Publishing Company, 2006.

Graham, Douglas N. *The High Energy Diet Recipe Guide.* Key Largo, FL: Douglas N. Graham, 2003.

Howell, Edward. *Enzyme Nutrition: The Food Enzyme Concept.* Wayne, NJ: Avery Publishing Group, 1985.

Kenney, Matthew, and Sarma Melngailis. *Raw Food / Real World: 100 Recipes to Get the Glow.* New York: HarperCollins, 2005.

Kirschmann, John D., with Lavon J. Dunne. *Nutrition Almanac,* second edition. New York: McGraw-Hill, 1984.

Kulvinskas, Viktoras. *Love Your Body: Live Food Recipes.* Woodstock Valley, CT: Omangod Press, 1972.

Malkmus, George H., with Peter and Stowe Shockey. *The Hallelujah Diet.* Shippensburg, PA: Destiny Image Publishers, 2006.

Malkmus, George H., with Michael Dye. *God's Way to Ultimate Health: A Common Sense Guide for Eliminating Sickness Through Nutrition.* Shelby, NC: Hallelujah Acres Publishing, 1995.

Malkmus, Rhonda J. *Hallelujah Holiday Recipes from God's Garden.* Shelby, NC: Halleluhah Acres Publishing, 2005.

———. *Recipes For Life . . . from God's Garden.* Shelby, NC: Hallelujah Acres Publishing, 1998.

Markowitz, Elysa. *Living with Green Star: A Gourmet Collection of Living Food Recipes,* revised edition. Cerritos, CA: Choison Publishing Company, 1997.

Mars, Brigitte. *Rawsome!: Maximizing Health, Energy, and Culinary Delight with the Raw Foods Diet.* Laguna Beach, CA: Basic Health Publications, 2004.

McIntyre, Anne. *Drink to Your Health: Delicious Juices, Teas, Soups, and Smoothies That Help You Look and Feel Great.* New York: Fireside, 2000.

McKeith, Gillian. *You Are What You Eat: The Plan That Will Change Your Life.* New York: Plume, 2006.

Nearing, Helen. *Simple Food for the Good Life: Random Acts of Cooking and Pithy Quotations.* White River Junction, VT: Chelsea Green Publishing Company, 1980.

Nison, Paul. *The Raw Life: Becoming Natural in an Unnatural World,* fourth edition. West Palm Beach, FL: 343 Publishing Company, 2004.

Onstad, Dianne. *Whole Foods Companion: A Guide for Adventurous Cooks, Curious Shoppers, and Lovers of Natural Foods,* revised and expanded edition. White River Junction, VT: Chelsea Green Publishing, 2004.

Patenaude, Frederic. *Instant Raw Sensations: The Easiest, Simplest, Most Delicious Raw-Food Recipes Ever!* Montreal, Canada: Raw Vegan, 2005.

Rinzler, Carol Ann. *The Complete Book of Food: A Nutritional, Medical & Culinary Guide.* New York: World Almanac, 1987.

Robbins, John. *Diet for a New America.* Walpole, NH: Stillpoint Publishing, 1987.

Romano, Rita. *Dining in the Raw.* New York: Kensington Books, 1992.

Safron, Jeremy A. *The Raw Truth: The Art of Preparing Living Foods.* Berkeley, CA: Celestial Arts, 2003.

Santillo, Humbart. *Food Enzymes: The Missing Link to Radiant Health,* second edition. Prescott, AZ: Hohm Press, 1993.

———. *Intuitive Eating: Every Body's Natural Guide to Total Health and Lifegiving Vitality Through Food.* Prescott, AZ: Hohm Press, 1993.

Shannon, Nomi. *The Raw Gourmet.* Burnaby, BC, Canada: Alive Books, 1999.

Underkoffler, Renee Loux. *Living Cuisine: The Art and Spirit of Raw Foods.* New York: Avery, 2003.

Walker, N.W., D.Sc. *Become Younger.* Prescott, AZ: Norwalk Press, 1995.

Weil, Andrew. *Eating Well for Optimum Health: The Essential Guide to Bringing Health and Pleasure Back to Eating.* New York: HarperCollins Publishers, 2000.

Wigmore, Ann. *Recipes for Longer Life.* Wayne, NJ: Avery Publishing Group, Inc., 1978.

Wolfe, David. *Eating for Beauty.* San Diego, CA: Maul Brothers Publishing, 2002.

Wolfe, David, and Sharon Holdstock. *Naked Chocolate.* San Diego, CA: Maul Brothers Publishing, 2005.

Resources

Here are my favorite mail-order suppliers offering both commonly available and specialty raw snack recipe ingredients of absolutely superb quality. Also included are a couple of raw food educational Web sites that might be of particular interest to my readers.

Champlain Valley Apiaries
800-841-7334
www.champlainvalleyhoney.com
Raw honey, maple syrup, beeswax, beeswax candles, and bee pollen. This Web site offers information on honey and its nutritional benefits, as well.

Gold Mine Natural Food Co.
800-475-3663
www.goldminenaturalfoods.com
A wonderful company that caters to organic, macrobiotic, vegan, raw, and gluten-free lifestyles. It also carries cookware, cutlery, supplements, natural body and oral care products, and books.

Honey Gardens Apiaries, Inc.
802-877-6766
www.honeygardens.com
Supplier of fresh, raw honey, beeswax, beeswax candles, bee pollen, propolis healing salve, and delicious honey-herbal blend health-promoting syrups. This Web site is quite informational about honey and its uses for both health and medicine.

Jaffe Bros.
760-749-1133
www.organicfruitsandnuts.com
Specializes in dried fruits, raw almond butter, seeds, beans, nuts, flours, grains, olives, spices, cereals, organic oils, prepared foods, raw honey and agave nectar, bee pollen, and organic coffee.

Jean's Greens
888-845-8327
www.jeansgreens.com
A range of wonderful herb products, teas, loose herbs and spices, essential oils, packaging supplies, base oils, beeswax, butters, clays, books, and more.

King Arthur Flour— The Bakers Catalogue
800-827-6836
www.kingarthurflour.com
Fabulous flavorings, measuring tools, quality kitchen appliances and gadgets, seasonings, tasty flours, superb olive oil, and more.

Living Foods
www.living-foods.com
An Internet community dedicated to educating the world about the power of living and raw foods. This Web site contains lots of raw food recipes and interesting information.

Living Tree Community Foods
800-260-5534
www.livingtreecommunity.com
Retailer of awesome, organic nut butters, nuts, seeds, dried fruit, olives, and raw honey. Superb quality!

MtnHoney

www.mtnhoney.com

"Best Honey in the World"—winner of the 2005 World Honey Show and recipient of the "Best Tasting Honey Award" from *Food & Wine Magazine* 2008, it specializes in delicious, raw sourwood honey as well as wildflower honey.

Mountain Rose Herbs

800-879-3337

www.mountainroseherbs.com

Carries everything you could possibly want related to herbs, plus spices, raw cocoa, herb seeds, books, teas, essential and base oils, packaging supplies, herbal health aids, natural personal care products, and more.

Pines International, Inc.

800-697-4637

www.wheatgrass.com

Excellent source for organic wheatgrass, barley grass, alfalfa, beet juice, and whole food blend powders and tablets.

RawGuru, Inc.

800-577-4729

www.rawguru.com

Retailer of raw cocoa, raw foods, and kitchen equipment for the raw foodist. The Web site contains lots of raw food recipes and educational information.

Stephanie Tourles

www.stephanietourles.com

My Web site. Licensed holistic esthetician, author, herbal practitioner, certified aromatherapist, nutritionist, and raw food enthusiast!

Sunfood Nutrition

888-729-3663

www.sunfood.com

Offers raw foods, raw cocoa, nut butters, super foods and supplements, books, DVDs, body care products, and kitchen appliances for the raw foodist.

Sun Organic Farm

888-269-9888

www.sunorganic.com

Supplier of dried fruits, raw nuts, seeds, beans, grains, flours, raw nut butters, raw cocoa, organic coffee, spices, prepared foods, raw honey and agave nectar, bee pollen, and more.

Tribest Corporation

888-254-7336

www.tribestlife.com

Retailer of unique kitchen appliances and gadgets for the raw foodist, plus cutlery, raw foods, supplements, and books.

USDA National Agriculture Library

www.nal.usda.gov/afsic/pubs/csa/csa.shtml

The government's Web page on starting or finding a CSA farm.

Wood Prairie Farm

800-829-9765

www.woodprairie.com

A source for fresh organic vegetables and gourmet potatoes, plus beans, wheat berries, oat groats, spelt berries, whole grain cereals, bread mixes, sprouting seeds, organic cheese, dried fruit, and organic garden seeds. Nice folks from Maine!

Index

Page numbers in *italics* indicate photos.

Other Storey Titles You Will Enjoy

Healing Tonics
by Jeanine Pollak

Tasty, health-promoting recipes for drinks that can help boost
mental clarity, increase stamina, aid digestion, support heart health, and more.

160 pages. Paper. ISBN 978-1-58017-240-0.

Lift Me Up/Calm Me Down
by Stephanie Tourles & Barbara Heller

Dozens of fresh ideas and simple suggestions for gearing up or
cooling down — whatever the day demands.

480 pages. Paper. ISBN 978-1-58017-163-2.

Making & Using Dried Foods
by Phyllis Hobson

Step-by-step instructions for drying almost everything with or
without a commercial dehydrator.

192 pages. Paper. ISBN 978-0-88266-615-0.

Organic Body Care Recipes
by Stephanie Tourles

Homemade, herbal formulas for glowing skin, hair, and nails, plus a vibrant self.

384 pages. Paper. ISBN 978-1-58017-676-7.

Rosemary Gladstar's Herbal Recipes for Vibrant Health

A practical compendium of herbal lore and know-how for wellness,
longevity, and boundless energy.

408 pages. Paper. ISBN 978-1-60342-078-5.

These and other books from Storey Publishing are available
wherever quality books are sold or by calling 1-800-441-5700.
Visit us at www.storey.com.